'This book is the equivalent of inviting a very interesting and knowledgeable forensic psychologist round for dinner, and using the opportunity to pick their brains about the reality behind the tabloid headlines that scream out at us on the subject of violent or sexual crime. Stories (aka detailed case studies) are used to skilfully unravel psychological explanations for such acts. Make yourself a cup of tea, pull up a chair, and get ready to lose yourself in a fascinating read that will inspire, captivate, and educate, regardless of your starting level of knowledge. And you may as well cancel that newspaper subscription while you are at it – superficial headlines will simply annoy you hereafter.'

—*Belinda Winder, Nottingham Trent University, UK*

'*Forensic Case Histories* provides invaluable insight into the growing reliance on risk assessment in criminal justice. Craissati draws on her unparalleled experience to juxtapose individual case studies with wider research, making complex concepts accessible. It is essential reading for all professionals, lawyers, and judicial bodies working with people convicted of serious offences.'

—*Simon Creighton, Bhatt Murphy Solicitors, UK*

Forensic Case Histories

Forensic Case Histories: Understanding Serious Offending Behaviour in Men examines men's violent and sexual offending behaviours, outlined through a series of real offender narratives, from a psychological perspective and in an accessible manner that will engage any audience, from the criminology-intrigued layperson to the specialist in the field.

This unique and conversational text thinks psychologically about serious crime, offering a compilation of men's narratives that explore their life experiences and the ways in which these experiences influence their behaviour in adulthood. Each chapter addresses a particular theme, covering frequently asked questions in the field such as, 'How can an apparently motiveless offence have meaning?' and 'Is psychopathy a personality disorder, and why do we struggle to treat individuals with such traits?' The narratives of individuals who offend are central to the discussion, but the chapters each draw on the relevant facts from the research literature and highlight key learning points. Many chapters also feature 'Further Reading' sections to expand readers' knowledge.

Both educational and accessible, *Forensic Case Histories* will appeal not only to specialists but also to any layperson curious to understand more about criminal acts. It is especially valuable to students and instructors of criminal justice, mental health, and related fields.

Dr. Jackie Craissati MBE has more than 30 years of experience in forensic mental health and criminal justice services, and is the author of five books on the subject of men with sexual convictions, and the management of offenders with a diagnosis of personality disorder.

Forensic Case Histories

Understanding Serious Offending Behaviour in Men

JACKIE CRAISSATI

Routledge
Taylor & Francis Group
LONDON AND NEW YORK

First published 2021
by Routledge
2 Park Square, Milton Park, Abingdon, Oxon OX14 4RN

and by Routledge
52 Vanderbilt Avenue, New York, NY 10017

Routledge is an imprint of the Taylor & Francis Group, an informa business

British Library Cataloguing-in-Publication Data
A catalogue record for this book is available from the British Library

Library of Congress Cataloging-in-Publication Data
Names: Craissati, Jackie, author.
Title: Forensic case histories: understanding serious offending behaviour in men/Jackie Craissati.
Description: Abingdon, Oxon; New York, NY: Routledge, 2021. | Includes bibliographical references and index. |
Identifiers: LCCN 2020032926 (print) | LCCN 2020032927 (ebook) |
ISBN 9780367360832 (hardback) | ISBN 9780367360863 (paperback) |
ISBN 9780429343759 (ebook)
Subjects: LCSH: Sex offenders–Psychology–Case studies. | Sex offenders–Rehabilitation–Case studies. | Psychosexual disorders–Case studies. |
Criminal psychology–Case studies.
Classification: LCC RC560.S47 C735 2021 (print) | LCC RC560.S47 (ebook) |
DDC 616.85/83–dc23
LC record available at https://lccn.loc.gov/2020032926
LC ebook record available at https://lccn.loc.gov/2020032927

ISBN: 978-0-367-36083-2 (hbk)
ISBN: 978-0-367-36086-3 (pbk)
ISBN: 978-0-429-34375-9 (ebk)

Typeset in Dante and Avenir
by KnowledgeWorks Global Ltd.

Contents

Acknowledgements

I would like to express my gratitude and thanks to my loyal 'focus group' – Erin, Emma, Ian, Kay, Pauline, and Venu – who provided invaluable comments, criticisms, and insights on each of the chapters. I am indebted to you all.

About the author

Dr. Jackie Craissati MBE has more than 30 years of experience of working in forensic mental health and criminal justice services. Prior to setting up Psychological Approaches CIC with two fellow practitioners, she was Clinical Director of a large forensic and prison service in Oxleas NHS Foundation Trust, southeast London.

She is well known for overseeing the Challenge Project – a 25-year-long rolling group work programme for individuals with high-risk sexual convictions; she has also led the development of innovative community services for individuals with serious offending behaviour and a diagnosis of personality disorder, including partnerships with the voluntary sector. A strong advocate of clinically applied research, she is the author of 5 books and more than 40 journal publications.

1 Introduction

Setting the scene

Taking a curious approach

This is a book about stories, stories told through the lens of professional engagement with men who have committed serious acts of violence – physical and sexual – against others. It takes a narrative approach, by which I mean that the stories provide a detailed account of a series of linked events and personal experiences that culminate in an act of violence. The book assumes a curious approach in the reader; that is, it is written for those who feel the urge to know more, those who tend to be inquisitive and want to try and figure things out, particularly the peculiarities of human behaviour. The book may well satisfy those individuals who find themselves reading about serious crimes and – after the initial recoil of horror, the compassionate identification with the victim, and secret sigh of relief that it happened to someone else – can't resist wondering 'why did he do it?' A curious stance can be uncomfortable, but it is often a creative one, it opens up possibilities, new lines of inquiry, it avoids the trap of overgeneralising leading to false assumptions. Nevertheless, seriously violent acts challenge our moral compass – rightly so – and provoke us to rush to condemn the perpetrator. Many of us know someone – family, friend, or neighbour – who has suffered violence at the hands of another, and the affront can feel very personal indeed. It is for this reason that our initial response to a violent crime is often one of instant judgement; our approach is then to seek information that confirms our original hypothesis, and in so doing, provide comforting reassurance. This is sometimes called confirmation bias – the tendency to seek information and/or to interpret evidence in ways that fit with what we already believe. One common example of confirmation bias is exemplified by press coverage: in the summer of 2019 as I write this introductory chapter, a released life-sentenced prisoner, who absconded from his probation hostel and was at large for three months, has been caught and returned to prison. The reasons for his absconding and the fact that he apparently committed no new crime are irrelevant in terms of media coverage and public outrage; furthermore, the surprisingly low reoffending rate for those who reside in such hostels attracts no attention for this is not compatible with our deepest fears about individuals who have been violent. When teaching forensic psychology trainees, I often say that if you hear yourself saying 'don't you think that…', this should sound a personal alert! The nature of the phrase suggests you have a predetermined view, and have probably ceased to hold an open and curious mind about the mind of others.

This tension between our strong moral response and our curiosity is a challenge shared by all those who work professionally with individuals who have committed serious crimes. Over the course of training and the early years in work, we have to learn what to do with our emotional responses to the crime, whether to allow our moral outrage to remain in the room, or to risk personal compromise by leaving moral judgement outside the interview room door. The following snippet of dialogue between a psychologist and an individual serving a long-term sentence highlights the dilemma; the first extract is what I would call a morally driven interaction in response to a difficult but commonly encountered conversation about victims; the second is a curiosity-driven interaction; note the different outcomes.

PSYCHOLOGIST So tell me a bit about how you feel about the offence now, looking back.

INTERVIEWEE I know you want me to feel bad about it, but I don't, if the victim hadn't lied in court, I wouldn't have got this long sentence; she has a lot to answer for.

PSYCHOLOGIST What did the victim lie about?

INTERVIEWEE The rape, there was no rape; we had sex, yes, but she was the one who came on to me, she was willing.

PSYCHOLOGIST The court found you guilty of rape, and the victim statement clearly describes the way in which you forced her to have sex without her consent.

INTERVIEWEE Are you saying victims never lie? I can prove that the victim lied about a number of things. The court got it wrong, and that's all I have to say about it. I can see you don't believe me.

The psychologist has identified what we call 'cognitive distortions' (distorted thinking patterns) in the man who has been found guilty of rape. S/he is unambiguously and correctly identifying some of the inaccuracies in his account, and in doing so, shuts him down in terms of the interview. However, in this second snippet of dialogue, the psychologist ignores the distortions in favour of adopting a more curious and inquiring stance; without condoning the man's inaccurate blaming of the victim, s/he pursues an account of the offence from his perspective. That is, s/he suspended understandable moral responses, pushing them to the side (or out the door) whilst focusing on the individual in front of her.

PSYCHOLOGIST So tell me a bit about how you feel about the offence now, looking back.

INTERVIEWEE I know you want me to feel bad about it, but I don't, if the victim hadn't lied in court, I wouldn't have got this long sentence; she has a lot to answer for.

PSYCHOLOGIST Lie is a strong word, tell me a bit more about what you mean by it.

INTERVIEWEE We had sex, yes, but she was the one who came on to me, she was willing. There was no rape, she just changed her tune when her boyfriend found out what she'd been up to.

PSYCHOLOGIST Ok, so let's start at an earlier point when things were going well that evening; it sounds like you're pretty sure she was coming on to you at the start.... [T]ell me a bit more about how you met, and what you thought about her at that point.

INTERVIEWEE We met in the club, I'd seen her around before; she was pretty wild, drunk, but friendly, flirty. We got on ok, and I thought 'I'm in with a chance'.

In other words, professionals learn to adopt a curious approach that starts from the offender's perspective, in order to begin to understand why the offence happened. The fact that his perspective bears no resemblance to the victim's reality has to be held in mind but left unsaid for the time being. It is as if the perpetrator is on one side of a large wall, and we are on the other side, the side where the victim is located; we can try ordering the perpetrator to come over to our side of the wall, but this is unlikely to work if the perpetrator cannot or will not find a way across. We will have to find the right spot to cross – perhaps a weak point where the brickwork is crumbling, or where there are possible footholds to climb over; we have to show the perpetrator where to cross, and we may even have to cross over to his side in order to bring him back with us. These ideas about perpetrator and victim perspectives are returned to throughout this book, and we return to the victim issues later in this chapter.

Psychologically informed

The stories in this book are psychologically informed; that is, they are narrated in a way that is driven by psychological theories and knowledge. Psychology is the scientific study of the human mind and the ways in which it influences our behaviour; it can encompass diverse areas such as development, personality, motivation, thought processes, and emotions. When thinking about the world of offending, psychological theories tend to focus particularly on thinking and emotion in relation to behaviours (violent acts) that are thought to be 'abnormal' or 'problematic', outside the range of normal or usual human experience. Immediately this begins to pose problems, for it suggests a clarity of definition that bears little resemblance to reality. Right and wrong, rational and irrational may seem absolute concepts, but of course, our thinking shifts over time and place – social, cultural, and political contexts greatly influence our conceptions of 'abnormal'. As just one particularly stark example, homosexuality was illegal only 50 or so years ago; associated with this, there has also been a long tradition of individuals with a homosexual orientation being labelled as 'sexually deviant' and sent for psychological therapy with the aim of changing their sexual preferences. Shocking as this may seem to us now, it has been social change rather than psychological theory that has driven our approach to labelling sexual orientation as either 'normal' or 'abnormal'. Psychologists are also rightly criticised for being overly focused on the individual and his/her interpersonal relationships, pathologising (or medicalising) undesirable human behaviours; they have been accused of failing to focus sufficiently on the social drivers of criminal acts, such as poverty, gender, social class, stigma, and difference. Criminology – an offshoot of sociology – offers a view of offending that is rooted more in social theories, a perspective that is – I would argue – complementary to, rather than in competition with, a psychological approach. In a rather simplistic way, the relationship between a psychological and a sociological approach could be thought of as follows: social theories provide an invaluable cultural and political context in which to understand criminal behaviour, while psychological theories facilitate a more individualised understanding of why a particular individual committed a particular act at the time that he did. For example, we recognise domestic violence as a social issue, and some might argue convincingly that its current prevalence is related to patriarchal societies that invest power and control with men, and implicitly or explicitly endorse derogatory attitudes towards women. Nevertheless, psychological theories facilitate a more detailed understanding of why only a particular subgroup of men perpetrate violence on their partners, and specifically, how we might try to make sense of the extremes of 'abnormal' behaviours by intimate partners against women – stalking and homicide, for example – that challenge our ability to make sense of such behaviour.[1]

Psychology is a social science, and as such it adopts a rigorous academic approach to the development of theoretical ideas; hypotheses have to be tested – whether this entails clinical observations, the gathering of factual data, or both – before we can make assertions with some confidence. As with the natural sciences, our understanding mutates and evolves as we come to understand more about the human mind and behaviour, and theories have to be adjusted. The common assertion that psychology is mere 'common sense' has some truth to it, but can also be misleading. The fact is that we all have the capacity to recognise psychologically meaningful 'truths', as we go about our everyday lives: if you have ever noticed any of the following, you are operating as a psychologically informed observer, even if you do not fully understand the psychological theory underpinning your understanding:

- You notice you are repeatedly attracted to intimate partners who share similar traits and – unnervingly –these traits are not dissimilar to those of your father.
- Your friend is annoyingly clingy and possessive, but you recognise that this is probably because she feels insecure as a result of struggling to make friendships when you were at school together.
- You are trying to give up alcohol, but you tend to relapse into heavy drinking when you feel low in mood and lonely. You've noticed a regular pattern: after lapsing into one drink, you binge drink, telling yourself that you might as well as you've failed miserably, and you can start again the next day. Unfortunately, the next day you feel really low, and so the cycle continues.
- You know you have a bad temper, which you try hard to keep under control; very occasionally you have the unpleasant sensation of a 'red mist' coming over you, and later a vague memory of screaming at someone uncontrollably. It feels unreal at the time, almost as though you were watching yourself acting in a film.

However, not all psychological knowledge is drawn from a common sense interpretation of the world around us, and throughout this book, the case histories contain accounts that are counter-intuitive and that challenge our thinking. As already intimated, we may recognise impulses in ourselves that might be shared with individuals who have committed serious violent offences; for instance, all the examples above might also be observed as relevant to some offending behaviour. However, for most of us who have not offended, our behaviour has not spilled over into destructive acts of harm; this is sometimes described as not having breached the body barrier, a term used to highlight the significant step from thinking and feeling in relation to violence to acting on such thoughts and feelings. Research and inquiry is therefore key if we are to take our psychological understanding of offending to the next level; our experience alone is insufficient as evidence. There are many methodologies for psychological research, including in-depth interviews that seek emerging themes; questionnaire and survey approaches that elicit self-reported views; and large databases of individuals with their 'factual' characteristics recorded, which seek to determine significant links between this data and outcomes that could not be found by chance alone. This book is intended to be evidence-based and educational, anchored in an academic understanding that nevertheless intends to be accessible to a non-specialist reader. This means that the theoretical and clinical ideas put forward in the chapters would be considered to be sound and fairly mainstream by professional peers. It should be noted that there is probably a published research paper to endorse every possible variation of outcome or finding; the research relied on in this book is solely focused on robust findings. By robust, I mean research that is based on large samples of data, or that has been replicated more than once, with similar findings; that is, findings that are sound. For the interested reader and the student or trainee, references to useful facts and key research findings are signposted throughout the chapters and further reading is suggested at the end of each chapter.

Who are the men in the case histories?

This book focuses on men quite simply because men account for the vast majority of serious sexual and violent crimes. The case histories are, to some extent, representative of the wider group of individuals who are incarcerated for similar crimes, albeit that everyone has their own unique story to tell. This is not a book for those seeking the excitement of tales of serial killers or of those who have a certain notoriety having been in the public eye. Salacious curiosity – inquisitiveness that is driven by a desire for excitement rather than understanding – thrives on the unique and monstrous, the sense of 'other' in the perpetrator. The stories articulated in this book are those belonging to fairly ordinary people, individuals who have usually experienced rather difficult – sometimes traumatic – times; with hindsight their lives have taken a rather indirect route towards offending, with missed opportunities, bad luck, and poor decision-making littering the path; they are marked by the nature of their terrible destructive acts, but behind these acts, the men are recognisably like us – mundane to some extent, lonely, angry, hurt, or vengeful. There is never much glamour attached to such difficult lives.

The stories are drawn from my work with prisoners who are seeking to be heard by a Parole Board panel in relation to progression through prison into the community, or from those individuals I have seen as outpatients in my clinic, after their release into the community from prison or secure hospital. Some I have met on only one or two occasions over the past 30 years; others I have known for more than a decade; all have shared their stories with me, have seen what I have written about them, and have reflected on their learning and my observations regarding the meaning of their offending and the risk that they might pose to others. I have not drawn on any stories from men who have objected strongly to my assessment findings or to seeing me as an outpatient. Nevertheless, it has been extremely important to me to maintain a robust level of confidentiality with the case histories in this book; not only out of respect for the large number of men who have talked with me about their lives and their offending, but out of concern for their families and for the victims of their crimes. The stories are therefore all derived from the combined narratives of at least three individuals, with key details about the offences, the victims, and the background histories all changed and intermingled. Age, gender, dates, weapon type, and so on have all been altered whilst striving to retain the integrity of the individuals' core narrative. Here and there I have taken snippets of dialogue from actual conversations with individuals in order to illustrate a particular frame of mind, but these are heavily disguised within the altered narrative. It is my assertion that this heavy disguising of the stories does not dilute the psychological meaning of the narratives – although each individual is unique, he also shares a very similar set of responses to his peers with similar experiences; it is these thematic elements that are captured within the case histories.

Where does this leave the victims?

This chapter has already touched on the notion that there are a number of realities or truths to the narratives around serious violent crime: there is the perspective of the perpetrator who has an account not only of his role within the offence, but also an imagined reality regarding the victim's experience. To illustrate what I mean by this, if we re-read the brief extract of dialogue between the psychologist and the interviewee (see above) who had raped a woman, we have an inkling that the perpetrator has a personal narrative about what happened, but he also has a story in his mind about the victim's intentions – entirely from his own perspective of course. For the victim of a serious violent crime, the narrative and perspective may overlap with that of the perpetrator, but more often than not, the victim's experience will bear little resemblance to the perpetrator's story. Not only will the victim (or in the case of a killing, the victim's family) have been overwhelmed with incredibly difficult feelings at the time of the offence – feelings of terror, anger, or humiliation, as examples – but they may also construct a narrative about the perpetrator – that he intended to kill them, that he targeted them specifically, or that he is fundamentally evil – that does not match with our experience of the individual perpetrator many years later.

It seems to me that it is partly for this reason that retrospective narratives about an individual perpetrator's life experience can perhaps feel like a betrayal to a victim, a way of denying the validity of his/her experience of an attack. It can take many years for an individual to construct a meaningful narrative of his pathway to violence, and it is all too easy for a compassionate and empathic understanding of his difficulties to end up seeming like an excuse for an act that may well have scarred the victim for life. For victims of serious violent crime, this book may therefore feel too painful, too one-sided, too understanding of the perpetrator's perspective. The victims in this book are rather shadowy figures, two-dimensional in some ways, and very much thought about in terms of how the victim featured in the perpetrator's mind. For some victims, I like to think that understanding the perpetrator better may be helpful, but the reality is that it is probably more likely to be hurtful. It is for this reason that few professionals work with both victims and perpetrators of crime; the collision of emotions is too strong to handle without losing professional equilibrium. Put simply, working with victims makes one feel too angry with the perpetrators to be able to properly explore the latter's difficulties without judgement. However, there is also the danger that working with perpetrators pushes us into a collusive stance with the perpetrator's perspective that means we minimise, distort, and invalidate the enormity of the victim's experience. When working with individuals who have committed serious interpersonal violence, we try to solve this dilemma by holding the victim in mind, but at arm's length. By this I mean that as practitioners, we never rely solely on the perpetrator's self-report, but we read documents that represent the victim without overwhelming us with the victim's pain. Such documents include witness statements and the summing-up by judges at the end of a trial; they may also include probation reports completed shortly after conviction and victim statements at the time of a Parole Board hearing.

How the chapters have been structured

Each chapter is centred on a case history – sometimes on more than one individual – and is based around a theme. These themes have emerged over the course of many conversations with colleagues, students, and friends; they could be thought of as 'frequently asked questions', or habitual queries to key forensic conundrums. The case history or histories explore the key chapter theme, and then essential facts, important research findings, and key theoretical points are highlighted in boxes. Chapter 2 introduces the idea of an explanatory narrative in response to those who ask 'how can what happened to him as a child be related to his offence?' The idea of a psychologically informed narrative is central to the book, and this chapter focuses on the role of attachment theory to help us understand problems in the pathway to offending. Chapter 3 focuses on the thorny issue of denial, and explores a story in order to answer the question: 'surely if you deny your offence that means you're still risky?' Chapter 4 looks at the story of men who have offended after leaving the care system as a child, and tries to identify 'why so many children in care end up in the criminal justice system?' Chapter 5 considers men who sexually offend against children and who have themselves been sexually abused when a child; it seeks to answer the question: 'most people who are abused don't go on to abuse others, isn't it just an excuse?' Chapter 6 reveals the science behind risk assessment, and explores the risk profiles of two violent individuals. Chapter 7 focuses on the controversial label of personality disorder and psychopathy, and explores narratives that highlight the way in which problematic traits can contribute to offending. Chapter 8 examines the question of responsibility for serious offending for those with severe mental illness, drawing upon four case histories to describe the variable nature of the relationship between the offence and the mental disorder. Chapter 9 is about fantasy and the world of sexual and violent imagery; it tries to explain the counter-intuitive evidence as to whether such media/imagery fuels the likelihood of violent offending.

Chapter 10 is a little different. I talked earlier in this chapter about our moral compass, and the emotional responses that we, as professionals, may experience when sharing a therapeutic space with men who have committed serious acts of violence. Staying attuned to our emotional responses – as long as they do not overwhelm our capacity to think – is an important component of working therapeutically with an individual. Noticing discomfort, sadness, anger, boredom in ourselves, these observations can be thought of as a barometer of the working relationship. However, no matter how experienced a professional is, sometimes these emotions overwhelm our capacity to think clearly and spill out into the session. Chapter 10 focuses on my own experiences of these 'spillages' over the years, and examines times when I have struggled to manage difficult feelings in the sessions, and how these moments might be linked to the individual stories that I have been trying to make sense of.

Summary

This is a book about understanding men who have seriously harmed others, and who have been caught and punished through the Criminal Justice System. Drawing on psychologically informed perspectives, the book aims to explore the men's pathway to offending and the choices they made. The pathway to offending is rarely if ever predetermined: biology and genetics (our inherent traits) interact with our life experiences and the quality of our developing relationships and are strongly influenced by the social context in which individuals live their lives. Although each individual man's life story is personal and unique, there are commonalities in terms of their pathway into offending: key life choices are made at pivotal moments – usually in constrained circumstances with restricted opportunities – and apparently chance events interweave with habitual patterns of problematic behaviour to culminate in destructive acts. The narratives in this book are retrospective; they comprise a collaborative approach – the individual who has offended and the practitioner working with him – to making sense of those destructive acts.

Note

1. While I acknowledge that women can be perpetrators of domestic violence, this is a book that focuses on men who have offended, and therefore my examples are all similarly oriented towards male perpetrators.

2 Adam's story

Revealing the layers of meaning in an offence

In 1986, Adam stabbed and killed his wife from whom he was separated at the time. He received a mandatory life sentence, with a tariff of 15 years. This means that he needed to serve 15 years as the 'punishment' component of his life sentence, before he could be considered by the Parole Board for release; thereafter, the role of the Parole Board was to determine whether the risk of violence that Adam might pose to others was very low, such that he could be considered for release into the community. I met Adam 25 years after his original conviction and prior to his fourth Parole hearing, when he was again hoping to persuade the Parole Board panel that he had worked sufficiently hard to reduce his risk to a minimal level. My report concluded with the following analysis of Adam:

> *Adam's childhood development provides information that helps to understand the psychological drivers underpinning his offence. At an early age, his mother became severely mentally unwell and was erratic in her care of him; he experienced his father as inexplicably cold and rejecting towards him, and these experiences interfered with his ability to achieve a strong attachment to a secure nurturing carer. However, for a period of time, placed in the care of a loving aunt and uncle, Adam flourished, and any early emotional damage seemed to have been repaired. Tragically, as Adam was entering into adolescence, with the sudden illness of his uncle and the death of his aunt, he was again wrenched back to the emotionally impoverished environment of the parental home. This marked the beginning of a sustained period of 'acting out' behaviour in which he seems to have channelled feelings of anger into destructive – albeit rather petty – antisocial acts. In early adulthood, Adam met and married his wife, and with this emerged signs of developing*

> *maturity. Nevertheless, with the benefit of hindsight, one can see that he was dependent on his wife, but also not emotionally available to her, largely because – in my view – he feared abandonment. Ultimately, Adam's persistent heavy drinking triggered the final request by his wife for a divorce; I would suggest that it was the subsequent realisation that reconciliation was not a possibility, which triggered an extreme emotional reaction in him that had links to his two previous experiences of loss. He became utterly preoccupied with the need to possess his wife (alive or dead), rather than contemplate the possibility of rejection.*

The question is how did I arrive at this psychologically oriented 'explanation' of why the offence occurred? Psychologists often call this kind of summary a formulation: a formulation is framework for producing a narrative that explains the underlying cause or nature of the presenting problem (in this case, the offence of killing), linking this narrative to psychological theories. Ultimately – although not described above in terms of Adam – a formulation can enable us to generate some ideas about what sort of interventions or management might then resolve the difficulties identified in the formulation.

This chapter focuses on some of the general principles involved in approaching the task of understanding the meaning or function of offending behaviour from a psychological point of view. Although Adam's story is one of domestic homicide, these principles are relevant to most offences relating to interpersonal violence, sexual or physical. As individual case histories become more complex, we need to delve deeper into the possible layers of meaning underpinning apparently unreasonable and destructive acts of violence. In order to do this, it is important to understand a few fundamental concepts related to child development, most particularly the role of attachment in our emotional development; this chapter will explore attachment theory, and its relevance to thinking about interpersonal violence as a 'relational crime' (an idea that will be explained later in the chapter).

However, initially it is important to step back and start with the simplest of ideas – motive. A number of case histories presented in this book will have been described as 'motiveless crimes' – indeed, Adam's was reported as such by the media at the time. From a psychological point of view, there is almost certainly no such thing as a crime without motive; when people describe a crime as 'motiveless', they really seem to be saying that the crime does not have a motive that is immediately apparent, or a motive that appears to contain sufficient rationality or intensity to account for the enormity of the act that has been perpetrated.

Although my summary of 'formulation' to account for Adam's offence appears to be fairly complex, there is a legitimate point of view to assert that there is a very limited and much more simple range of human motives that account for offending behaviour, particularly offences of interpersonal violence. Searching the internet yields a number of models for crime motives: for example, a common assertion is that motive falls into three categories – financial greed, sexual or relational lust, and the pursuit of power. Other models, such as that proposed by the Centre for Crime and Justice,[1] cite the four L's – lust, love, loathing, and loot – as the core motives for murder. Yet such a simple thematic approach to understanding motives for violent crimes does not satisfy as an explanation; it fails to capture the infinite variation in human experience: the nuances of situations in which individuals might express their needs, seek connection to others, hate, despair, and – ultimately – destroy. Crime fiction, for example, finds endless means of creating apparently unique characters and plots based simply on the four L's; as a starting point, a search of the term 'murder mysteries' yielded 54 million results on the internet!

Detective novels are actually an excellent way of beginning to understand how a psychologically informed case history can be developed, with the psychologist as a kind of detective of the mind. Let us take Agatha Christie murder mysteries simply as an example of a familiar approach to detective story development, plucking two of the more well-known novels – *Murder on the Orient Express* and *The A.B.C. Murders*. We can see that Ms Christie has woven intricate plots around two of the four L's – loathing in terms of *Murder on the Orient Express*, and loot in terms of *The A.B.C. Murders*. Yet, of course, the novels only come to life and have meaning for the reader when the author develops the narrative with the following components (albeit often sequenced differently for dramatic effect):

- Setting the scene by introducing the key players in the narrative, including their most notable characteristics, locating the setting and the build-up – including a number of triggering events – to the murder.
- Describing the death of the victim (and/or the act of killing) with an analysis of the crime scene and the clues that may shed light on the motives of the perpetrator.
- An elaboration of the key players in terms of their personal history, the quality of their relationship with each other, and the emerging details of complexities in their life experience.
- The denouement, in terms of the identification of the murderer, with a compelling explanatory account that makes sense of all that has gone before.

BOX 2.1

A few facts

A Home Office Domestic Homicide Review (DHR) report (2016) examined the details of all DHRs over the course of one year and found that there were 33 homicides of intimate partners, two thirds of whom had a history of violence (half of whom were violent to the victim only, the other half being more generally violent to others); a knife was the weapon most commonly used, the killing mostly took place in the home; depression was diagnosed in two thirds of the intimate partner homicides, and it was very common that mental health problems and substance misuse co-occurred in the same perpetrators. More recent figures from the Office for National Statistics (2017/18) found that a third of women (63 out of 190) were killed by their partner or ex-partner – as compared to only 1% (7) of men. More generally, reports clearly emphasise separation as a key time of risk for women; although figures vary, perhaps as many as half of all such homicides occurring within a year of separation.

We can take this approach to the development of Adam's story – and do so later in this chapter – but before we follow the sequence set out so clearly by the Agatha Christie novels, it is important to pause and check the evidence base; that is, what might be known and published about domestic homicide – the term used when a victim is killed by someone to whom they are related, or who is a member of the same household, or with whom they had an intimate personal relationship. A psychologically informed approach means that the known evidence base provides an important baseline or context within which an individual's case history should be located. A huge amount has been written about domestic violence, including the identification of individuals whose violent behaviour within an intimate relationship escalates over time to the point of killing. However, much less has been written about those perpetrators – such as Adam – who were never known to be violent within the relationship; selfish, immature, feckless, and uncaring, but never violent. Box 2.1[2] highlights just a few facts about domestic violence, to set the scene, but these facts do not, in themselves, take us very far in understanding what happened in Adam's story.

Adam's story revisited

It is important to remember that I was meeting Adam 25 years after he had committed the offence of murder; his story had been shaped by the shock of the offence and his subsequent imprisonment, by personal reflection, gradual maturity, and the effects of a number of prison interventions. He repeatedly emphasised that he was no longer the person that he had been, and he spoke of his former self with something akin to despair and exasperation. He was a likeable man, of around average intelligence but not very verbally fluent when trying to express complex emotions. There was something rather engaging in the enthusiasm with which he spoke of his increasing self-awareness, although it was clear that he still struggled not to respond with excessive sensitivity if he felt himself to be criticised. This propensity to take offence had been a problem for him over the years in prison, and he had often locked horns with those in authority, retreating back into a stubborn stand-off when he felt that his efforts to change had been misunderstood or undervalued.

As intimated in the summary (or formulation) presented at the start to this chapter, the immediate context for the murder of his ex-wife was her understandable exasperation at his ongoing heavy drinking, and her decision to pursue a separation. Adam was able to recognise that he had been a poor husband, selfish in his habits, often out with friends, and a limited provider in terms of both money and affection. At the time, he simply could not believe that she would go ahead with the divorce, until the legal papers arrived one day in the post; this provoked him into a rage, and he went back to the house to confront her, they argued, he shoved her against the wall, and left. His ex-wife sought an injunction against him as a result, and this triggered a period of decline in Adam over about six weeks. His drinking became heavier, his sleep was poor, and he spent hours brooding upon his wife's 'unreasonable behaviour', either alone in his bedsit or sitting in his car outside the family home. Having never previously been a particularly jealous or possessive person, he found himself preoccupied with the possibility of her having an affair. In hindsight, it seems reasonable to conclude that Adam was becoming depressed in response to the breakdown of his marriage, but at the time he was unable to recognise this. Never one to open up about his feelings, Adam's communication with others was restricted to drinking pals with whom he exchanged little more than vague threats that *'she can't do this to me'*.

Adam has thought long and hard as to when the idea or the plan to hurt or kill his wife first came into his head and, of course, now we – and even he – will probably never be entirely sure. What does seem to be the case is that on the night of the murder, his thinking had already shifted from *'she can't do this to me'*, to *'I won't let her do this to me'*, and from *'I can't live without her'*, to *'she can't live without me'*. He was aware of a sense of inevitable and impending catastrophe, although he could not articulate this at the time other than in vague thoughts of *'it's either her or me'*. With these disturbed thoughts in his head, he left the pub and went to sit outside the house in his car, and it was chance that he happened to see a man leave the house (just a neighbour liaising with his wife about the garden fence); Adam was probably telling the truth when he said that he got out of the car with a surge of jealous fury, with no clear intent in mind other than to confront his wife – *'I think I knew that violence would happen, but not that I would kill her'*. It was when he let himself in by the kitchen door that he picked up a sharp knife from the drawer and then stabbed his wife a number of times as she came into the kitchen to see who was there.

The question now is whether we have enough information to say that we understand the offence. After all, Adam fulfilled a number of criteria associated with domestic homicides: he was intoxicated with alcohol and therefore disinhibited; his wife was divorcing him; he was jealous and angry; he had access to a knife. However, it is also the case that although women are much more likely to be murdered by their intimate partners than by anyone else, most estranged men do not attack their ex-partners, let alone kill them. Most men (and women of course) in such a situation will manage their intense emotional distress to a greater or lesser extent without hurting others; some might behave badly or seek help to get them through a difficult time, others might hold on to feelings of bitterness and resentment that colour their attitude to future relationships; some might wonder whether they will be able to cope, and possibly harbour, fleeting suicidal thoughts. To really understand Adam and his offence, we have to ask ourselves why he could not do this, was there some meaning for him in his wife's behaviour that went deeper than her understandable rejection of an unsatisfactory marriage. We need to ask ourselves why – in effect – he felt he had to destroy his wife in order to be able to go on with his life.

These questions go to the heart of the title of this chapter: revealing the layers of meaning in an offence. Sexual and violent offences can be thought of as relational crimes; by this I mean that in the perpetrator's mind, there is some kind of relationship with the victim – *real, displaced,* or *symbolic* – that may well bear little resemblance to the experience of the victim. In all the case histories in this book, this idea of a relationship with the victim, however fleeting, is returned to again and again. By *real*, I mean someone like Adam, whose relation with his wife was largely based in reality – they had been intimate partners until shortly before the murder. A *displaced* relationship is one in which the perpetrator's feelings are located temporarily in the victim, but really belong to another person: for example, a rapist may hold on to feelings of rage and humiliation in response to his mother's treatment of him as a child, and this is then re-experienced in relation to his recent girlfriend who has betrayed his trust by sleeping with another man; this anger is then acted upon and inflicted upon another when he brutally rapes a young female stranger who is walking home at night. A *symbolic* relationship is one in which the victim represents – for the perpetrator – a person or group of persons: for example, a prisoner, who fashions a lethal weapon in his cell and then attacks a prison officer who he feels is bullying him, may believe that he is taking revenge for all those in authority over him (his violent father, the disinterested teachers at school, the callous staff when he was in care) who have abused their position of trust.

In order to understand what Adam's existential dilemma on that night of the murder really means, we have to follow the clues that lie in his early life, and in his childhood development – that is, early experiences that shaped the way in which he understood the world, and the way in which he related to others (and expected others to relate to him). This is not to say that the murder was predetermined from an early age; simply that the template for how we relate to others is shaped by early experiences, and then repeatedly revised and reworked until we find ourselves in adulthood engaging in repeated patterns of interpersonal behaviour.

It is important to start by noting that, most commonly, there is little corroborative information available to support an individual's account of his early life, although the documents that comprise the Parole Board dossier do often contain early reports written at the time of the conviction which can be illuminating. The following account is one that is from Adam's perspective; it is not necessarily the account that his family would have provided if asked, or that an independent observer would have noted. When individuals talk about early experiences of adversity and abuse, we know that there can be multiple perspectives, and that poor parenting, neglect, and abuse can be inflicted by individuals who themselves have had impoverished early experiences as children. This bias in developing the narrative does not matter when thinking psychologically about someone, as it is always the individual's personal experience and the sense he has made of this experience that truly matters.

In Adam's case, he experienced a difficult start in life, although he only learnt the details later when he was old enough to absorb the information. Within a year of his birth, his mother had become mentally ill, a 'nervous breakdown' that she attributed to the strain of 'caring for Adam who was an unrewarding, screaming infant'. He could not recall these very early years, although we can surmise that his mother's behaviour was probably rather erratic and unpredictable, and that it was difficult for her to forge a strong and consistent bond with her baby boy; these days we might also wonder whether she was suffering from post-natal depression. Adam's father was disinterested in his baby son, and responded to Adam over the years usually with a distant coldness, and occasionally with a contemptuous and critical response to something that he had done. Around the age of 5, his parents handed him over to his mother's sister and her husband, who were a childless couple, and longing to care for him. Adam's experience was immediately transformed, and as a rather indulged only child, he quickly settled and formed local friendships. There was probably always a feeling in the back of his mind that his parents had not wanted him or loved him, and this was exacerbated by the arrival of his baby brother some five years later – a child that was the apple of his mother's eye, and close to his father who adored him. However, these insecurities and resentments were masked by the loving attention he received from his aunt and uncle.

As is so often the case when we delve into the narratives of individuals who have eventually committed serious violent offences, luck – or the lack of it – can often play a part in setting a new direction for the pathway to offending. In Adam's case, what appeared to be the reparation of early deprivation was abruptly terminated with the sudden death of his aunt from a stroke, and the subsequent decline in the health of his uncle who was no longer able to care for him. Perhaps if this tragic change in circumstances had occurred a few years later, he might have been better able to cope; but at the age of 10, he was suddenly returned to the care of his unwilling parents, cut off from his friendship group, pulled out of school, and living in a rather hostile environment. His parents chose – according to Adam – to deal with the situation by imposing strict boundaries and putting an end to any contact with his ailing uncle; a year later, when his uncle died, they felt it was unnecessary for him to attend the funeral. So it was a furiously angry and disoriented young boy who entered his adolescence, resentful and grieving, but with no means of articulating his feelings and no one to turn to.

Adam's adolescence was characterised by a deterioration in his behaviour at home and at school, particularly in terms of rather petty antisocial acts, including the destruction of property, petty theft, and – increasingly – disruptive drunken behaviour. In hindsight, Adam recognised that all of this behaviour was intended to annoy his parents and elicit a response from them. We call this 'acting out' – a term used to denote actions or behaviour that are undertaken rather than expressing the underlying emotions that are driving the behaviour. We are all prone to 'acting out'; for example, noting a doctor's appointment on the wrong day in the diary, and thereby missing the appointment, rather than allowing oneself to acknowledge or admit the fear associated with some rather worrying symptoms. Returning to Adam's situation, how interesting that his parents' indifference or apparent hostility to him was not matched by his own indifference to them. It was as if he felt compelled to prove that he mattered to them; 25 years later, Adam could also recall times when he really tried to seek his father's approval in a positive fashion – particularly when he got into the school football team – but the inevitable rejection was so painful that he reverted to the antisocial strategies that were less exposing of his vulnerability. This difficulty in achieving detachment and indifference is key to understanding the triggers for Adam's offence; in order to make sense of it, we need to understand attachment theory and why it matters.

Attachment theory and why it matters

The origins of attachment theory were first described by John Bowlby in the late 1960s, and this sparked decades of important research and theory development. It is important to understand the evolutionary premise that lies at the heart of the theory: children are thought to be born biologically pre-programmed to form attachments with others – particularly their key caregivers – in order to survive. As a species, humans are hugely vulnerable and dependent for many years, and rely on adults for protection; a threat to attachment (for example, abuse or neglect) is therefore responded to as a threat to survival, with the same fight-flight response as we might experience in response to a more tangible and physical threat.

In addition to this idea of security and survival, attachment – strong, consistent bonds with caregivers – enables infants to begin to develop important emotional and social skills. In simple terms, an early bond involves the caregiver:

- Tuning in and being responsive to the baby's emotional state
- Responding to such states with marked responses, including soothing mannerisms
- Introducing words that can symbolise or express the child's emotional state accurately

Repeated endlessly and with reasonable consistency, these are some of the means by which a child learns to develop a clear and positive sense of self, and an ability to label and manage their own emotional state as well as understanding the emotional states of others (something we might refer to as 'emotional intelligence'.

When bonding and attachment are problematic – for whatever reason – the infant/child experiences stress in line with the fight/flight response; we can all manage short periods of such stress, but prolonged insecurity or trauma in the attachment can lead to significant problems for the child in terms of feeling overwhelmed by negative emotional states, difficulty

BOX 2.2

Attachment theory

John Bowlby first used the term in the 1960s to describe the evolutionary imperative driving an infant's need to bond with a caregiver. That is, a strong emotional and physical attachment, consistently provided by a nurturing adult, is crucial to survival and personal development in humans.

retaining an ability to think when attachment systems are triggered, and chronic fears of abandonment associated with closeness to others.

We are now much clearer that attachments are more fluid and adaptive than previously thought. For example, we no longer believe that the mother provides the only or the crucial bond with a child; we also know that early adversity can be overcome with secure attachments being achieved later in childhood, and conversely, that early security in attachments can be damaged by later experiences in relating to others. Adolescence is a crucial time of opportunity – to repair early adversity in primary relationships – with both biological change (such as hormonal changes and brain development) and important new psychological and social tasks. To explain this latter point a little more, adolescence in western societies is thought of as a time when individuals pull away from their primary familial bonds and seek to develop their sense of self in relation to others via new attachments outside the family: with their peers in terms of friendships and sexual intimacy, and with social institutions. Those with positive and secure early attachment experiences are often – but not always – more resilient and able to cope with setbacks in this adolescent task; secure attachment acts as a buffer against later adversity. However, adolescence can also be a time of risk, when early adversity is consolidated by negative experiences and/or lack of opportunity to experience reparative attachments. That is, if an individual's early attachment experiences are insecure and associated with potential threat, then they are less resilient in the face of later adversity. In summary, although early attachment never predetermines the pathway into offending, for many of the individual narratives in this book, adolescence was a time in which early difficulties were aggravated rather than ameliorated.

Concluding Adam's narrative

Understanding the evolutionary imperative driving our attachment behaviours perhaps helps us to understand a little more about Adam's state of mind. We can see that his parents' early but sustained rejection of him was associated with a sense of personal threat to survival (at least unconsciously) that rendered him vulnerable in a number of ways: he lacked an emotional vocabulary with which to express his state of mind; rather understandably, he lacked resilience in coping with and processing his second loss of attachment figures; his sense of himself as an individual was precarious, and tended to be overly reliant on how others perceived him – and overly sensitive to their 'lack of approval'. In early adulthood, Adam threw himself impulsively into his marriage – perhaps a sign that he was trying to repair an earlier attachment vulnerability – but his behaviour was highly ambivalent. Such individuals long to be loved, and in return, to love another, but this longing is associated with a sense of fundamental threat – the terror of potential abandonment; sometimes it is easier to control the feared event – rejection – by triggering it, rather than to experience it at the whim of others. Adam's persistently unacceptable behaviour in his marriage pushed his wife to her limits, and in some ways, enabled Adam to force her rejection of him. The injunction and divorce papers that ensued were clearly strong symbolic markers of what he feared most – yet another experience of abandonment. For many, reading the story of Adam still requires a stretch of the imagination to understand why he then felt that his wife's rejection of him was a question of personal survival – 'her or me'. However, if we understand attachment as a fundamental prerequisite for our survival, and if we track the pathway to the offence via a series of failures to repair early attachment damage – some of which were simply 'bad luck' – then it becomes a little clearer as to why Adam's storm of wild and unthinking emotion at the time of the attack was experienced by him almost as form of psychic self-defence, although he would never have used those words.

Epilogue

Taking a curious and compassionate approach to understanding Adam's offence should not be confused with any form of soft-hearted justification for his behaviour. It took him years to face up to the enormity of his behaviour, and yet more years to develop a vocabulary with which to articulate a psychologically meaningful narrative. Post-tariff, four Parole Board panels remained unconvinced about his risk, until he was finally recommended for release. It was only when he was able to focus on relationships in the here and now – with prison and probation staff – that he was able to identify his need for approval and his sensitivity to perceived criticism; impasse turned gradually into dialogue, and dialogue gradually transformed into insight; finally, insight turned into a more consistent change in interpersonal behaviour patterns.

Notes

1. https://www.crimeandjustice.org.uk/sites/crimeandjustice.org.uk/files/09627250608553401.pdf
2. Home Office (2016). Domestic Homicide Reviews: Key Findings from Analysis of Domestic Homicide Reviews. https://assets.publishing.service.gov.uk/government/uploads/system/uploads/attachment_data/file/575232/HO-Domestic-Homicide-Review-Analysis-161206.pdf

Further reading

Reliable sources of statistics on particular crimes or particular types of offender can be difficult to find, and papers that have not been subject to peer review and scrutiny, or research based on small samples, are potentially misleading. **The Office of National Statistics** (www.ons.gov.uk) is the UK's largest independent producer of official statistics and is a reliable starting point. Within this website, the findings of the **Crime Survey for England and Wales** can be found; this is considered to be the 'gold standard' of crime surveys and far more indicative of the true crime rate than official police and court records.

In the United States, I suggest the **National Crime Victimization Survey** (https://www.bjs.gov), and recommend the material available from the **Office of Justice** (https://ojp.gov/).

There are a number of books written about formulation within a psychotherapeutic or a criminal justice setting. However, a good starting point for more information would be:

National Offender Management Service (2015). *Working with Offenders with Personality Disorder: A Practitioners Guide*, 2nd edition. https://www.gov.uk/government/publications/working-with-offenders-with-personality-disorder-a-practitioners-guide.

In terms of attachment theory, a very accessible book that provides quite sophisticated detail in a readable way is:

Gerhardt, S. (2015). *Why Love Matters: How Affection Shapes a Baby's Brain*. East Sussex: Routledge.

For more information on John Bowlby's work in the 1960s, see:

Bowlby J. (1969). *Attachment and Loss, Vol. 1: Attachment*. New York, NY: Basic Books.

Bill and Chris' story 3

Understanding why denying the offence might be a protective factor and unrelated to future risk

Bill's story

Bill was a 37-year-old self-employed computer software consultant when he was convicted of six counts of indecent assault on two young brothers who lived nearby. This was his first time ever before the court. He pleaded not guilty at trial, and although found guilty, he maintained his innocence for the first four years of his seven-year prison sentence. The assaults had taken place over a two-year period, at a time when the boys were rather unsettled and vulnerable as their parents were undergoing an acrimonious divorce. Bill – as friend and neighbour to the parents – was sometimes enlisted as an occasional babysitter; his relationship with the boys developed, and they were often found around at his house, playing computer games of which he had a thrilling supply. The indecent assaults – fondling and masturbation – developed over time, until the older brother eventually told a friend at school, who in turn told a teacher, and the police were called. Bill's elaborate explanation to the police and at the subsequent trial was that there had been one occasion when he was urinating in his toilet, and the older brother entered the room as Bill had forgotten to lock the door; he thought that maybe the boy had misunderstood his *'joke about there being enough room for two of us.... [W]e were just fooling about'*. Aside from that single incident, Bill maintained that the boys' account was entirely fictitious, probably developed as a means of *'gaining attention from their distracted parents who were neglecting them'*, although at times he hinted that it was conceivable that the boys' father may possibly have been inappropriate with them.

Bill was quiet and well-behaved during his sentence, but over time he was noted to become tearful and depressed, with some vague and fluctuating suicidal thoughts. The healthcare team – with his permission – referred him to the prison counselling service. Bill engaged well with his counsellor, and it was only after several sessions that he started to open up about his own experiences of being sexually abused by an uncle when a child; this step seemed to enable him to open up about his offending, and within a single session he suddenly blurted out a complete confession to everything the victims had alleged about him.

In later years, Bill had some interesting and rather articulate observations to make regarding his former stance of total denial: *'I felt that if I were to admit, it would be like destroying myself.... I know that sounds very dramatic, but it felt like it would be a catastrophe – everything that I was, or that I thought I was, would go, I would be nothing more than a pervert. ... Somehow, the fact that my few friends and my mum and sister believed in me – that I was innocent – kept me trapped in this world, and I had no means of escaping it. ... [N]ot that I'm sure I wanted to escape it, I was too much of a coward for that, it was convenient to hide behind my denial, my innocence, I could almost deny it to myself; it's amazing that there were times I really thought I hadn't done it. ... Over time, I knew it was eating away at me, it was like a growth inside me; and it became confused with what had happened to me as a child, so that I couldn't work out what I felt more ashamed about, or who had done what to whom. Madness I know. Telling the counsellor was actually a relief, a huge relief; but telling mum and my sister was so difficult. So I watered it down at first, just hints that something might have happened, that I was also a victim as a child, that I was depressed and wasn't fully in control of myself. ... You know, the sort of thing that tries to break the news gently. But nothing really makes something like child abuse sound ok; I don't think my mum has taken it in at all, she blames counselling for putting ideas in my head. My sister is more realistic about it, she kept asking me why, why, why? She hasn't spoken a word to me since, I don't think she ever will, she has kids and she feels I've betrayed her and the family, which of course I have. So it's a mixed blessing, but overall I feel better in myself even though I am more alone now than ever'.*

This is a chapter about a counter-intuitive idea – that denial of the offence might bear no relationship to the likelihood of an individual with a sexual conviction going on to commit a further sexual offence at some point in the future. Indeed, as the chapter title suggests, it is possible that the reasons underpinning this perplexing fact – and it is a robust and empirically driven fact – are actually protective in nature. If we link this to the account of Bill above, the natural assumption that most of us might make is that Bill's denial of the offence was a risk factor when considering the possibility of his release, and his subsequent admittance of all his sexual offending must have reduced his risk of future sexual offending. However, although Bill has done what we might consider to be a morally correct thing – even if a little late in the day – in admitting culpability, and he undoubtedly seems to feel more at ease with himself for doing so, it is the case that this confession, in itself, has not changed anything in terms of future risk. His account does – as does Chris's somewhat different account later in this chapter – raise questions as to what the function or meaning of denial might be for the perpetrator, and this chapter explores what we think is the explanation for its lack of link to risk.

At the time of arrest and trial, there are sound and rational reasons – albeit we might describe them as cowardly and immoral ones – for maintaining one's innocence if charged with a sexual offence. It is well documented that charges can falter at all stages in the legal process, and even if matters proceed to court, opportunities for plea bargaining can downgrade the seriousness of the final charge. No sensible person would wish to acquire a sexual conviction if it could be avoided; the evidence suggests that persistent denials can lead to 'better' outcomes for the alleged perpetrator. Uncomfortable as it is to admit, there are also a small number of unsafe convictions which are later overturned when new evidence is presented at appeal; that is, a small minority of convicted sex offenders are indeed likely to be innocent. The case library of the Criminal Cases Review Commission in the United Kingdom and the Innocence Project in the United States[1] highlight this small but significant group of individuals. However, on the assumption that very few perpetrators are wrongly convicted, from a psychological point of view, denial becomes more interesting the longer it persists post-conviction (when the reasons for sustaining denial diminish greatly); and our interest is most piqued when insisting on one's innocence seems to be more important than being considered for release back into the community, at which point the outcome of denial seems to be almost entirely self-destructive.

What do we mean by denial?

Denial is sometimes referred to as full (or total or absolute) denial and partial denial. The former is quite simply an assertion that he – whether Bill, Chris, or another – did not commit the offence at all. This tends to fall into three broad groups: those who say they were not there and have been mistaken for another perpetrator; those who simply say nothing happened; and those who say that the sexual encounter was consensual and therefore not an assault. Bill falls into the middle group, and Chris's story will clearly allocate him to the latter group. Studies tend to show that around 30% of

BOX 3.1

Denial

Denial can be differentiated into *total denial* ('I didn't do it') and *partial denial* (minimising and rationalising behaviour).

Partial denial can be for:

- The acts themselves
- Responsibility for the acts
- The impact of the behaviour

convicted sex offenders maintain total denial of their convictions; but there is a further 30% or so who maintain partial denial throughout their sentence, and it is to this group that we now turn. Partial denial of a sexual offence can also be referred to as minimisations or rationalisations – the cognitive distortions that were mentioned in Chapter 1. These tend to focus on one or more of three areas:

- **Partial denial of the acts themselves**. This is when a perpetrator admits to some of the assaults or some of the alleged behaviour, but denies other aspects, often the more serious allegations. It is very common for an individual, for example, to deny their rape conviction but admit their lesser sexual assault conviction.
- **Partial denial of responsibility for the behaviour**. This is when a perpetrator admits to the act, but allocates blame to a factor outside himself. Often, individuals place great emphasis on the role of alcohol intoxication in controlling their actions, or blame the alleged infidelity of an intimate partner, or being made redundant at work.
- **Partial denial of the impact of the behaviour**. This is when a perpetrator admits to the act, takes responsibility for his actions, but plays down the impact of his behaviour on the victim. Individuals who partially deny often refer to the sexual 'knowingness' of the victim, or her lack of physical struggle, 'she never said no', or point to a child's behaviour in accepting gifts in exchange for further abuse (something most of us would understand as psychological control and coercion).

It is not difficult to understand that the key mechanism behind these types of partial denial is to make the perpetrator feel less bad about what has occurred; the fact is that we all employ this mechanism of partial denial to avoid feeling bad about ourselves – whether it involves minimising how badly behaved we were when drunk, or blaming our friend's superb baking skills for breaking our strict diet.

Bill's story provides us with some more sophisticated clues as to what the function of denial might be. He describes rather vividly the threat that a sexual conviction posed to his sense of himself, a sense in which he simply could not incorporate the identity of 'sex offender' into his self-image without shattering everything that he thought he was. We also have an inkling that denial was important in preserving important links to others in his life; in other words, denial was important both for himself and also in terms of his attachments; that is, his family needed to share a belief in his innocence, in order to be able to accommodate the fact of his conviction.

The difference between guilt and shame: denial as a shame-avoiding strategy

Guilt is a feeling state, largely internally driven; an unpleasant personal awareness of wrongdoing or culpability – feeling bad – that often has the potential to evoke strong feelings of anxiety in us. It is helpful here to differentiate feelings of guilt from shame; the latter can be thought of as a social or moral emotion that can be evoked when a negative evaluation of the self is compared to the social standard. Put simply, a guilty secret can become shameful when it is exposed to the judgment of others. Let us consider an example that does not involve an illegal act, but a behaviour that most of us can imagine occurring within our social network: a woman conducts a sexual liaison with another man while she is cohabiting within a committed intimate relationship, and without her partner's consent – she is unfaithful. She feels guilty, as she knows full well that her behaviour is '*wrong*' or at the very least '*hurtful*' to her partner; however, whilst it remains a secret, she can manage her guilt sufficiently, at least to the extent that she does not bring the sexual liaison to an end. She engages in a range of minimising or justifying thinking strategies (as described above in relation to offenders); these might include convincing herself she will stop the affair soon, that her husband is neglectful and she is justified, or that sex is not meaningful like a relationship. However, let us imagine that the affair is discovered, and she is confronted by her partner. This confrontation provokes a whole new set of emotions in her, as she is forced to face her partner's anger and hurt; her guilty secret is exposed and subject to the judgement of others. She feels ashamed, and she suddenly feels anxious, as she is faced with the reality of her behaviour, her partner might leave her, what will her friends and family think about her behaviour? With this feeling of shame – the guilt exposed – she finds herself strenuously denying the affair, her partner is *'mistaken'*, he has *'misinterpreted her behaviour'*, there is *'nothing to be concerned about'*; and temporarily, her anxiety is assuaged, she almost persuades herself in that moment that she is the wronged one in the partnership. Although you may protest that this woman is unusual in her dishonest denial of her behaviour, a number of published surveys of infidelity within intimate relationships suggest that the majority of those who have affairs never tell their partners, and of the minority who are found out, only a small percentage admit the affair. That is, in general terms, most of us in her position would feel a strong impulse to respond as she did.

If we return to our consideration of the link between denial and offending behaviour, the theoretical explanation is laid out in Box 3.2. Denial is a commonly used strategy to avoid the negative feelings of anxiety and humiliation associated with the shameful exposure of our guilt. In the example above, we examined a behaviour that may be frowned upon by many, but is neither illegal nor violent. If we then consider the most socially abhorrent of crimes – sexual offences – it becomes possible to imagine why denial can become so entrenched a response to try and fend off the devastation of an individual's sense of self. Indeed, we have an indication of just how ashamed individuals feel when their sexual offending comes to light: a systematic review of studies into suicide linked to arrest for a sexual offence found that such individuals were approximately 200 times more likely to take their life than someone in the general population, the highest risk period being 48 hours to one month after an investigation into the sexual offence has commenced. It is reasonable to conclude that stigma and shame were likely to be driving factors in this risk to self.

BOX 3.2

Guilt, shame, and denial

GUILT: a feeling of having committed a wrong, which induces a sense of anxiety

SHAME: a painful feeling of humiliation or distress caused by the exposure of wrongdoing

DENIAL: a healthy – albeit immature – response to manage the uncomfortable level of anxiety provoked by the humiliating shame of exposure to others as a sex offender

Chris's story

Before examining issues of denial and risk further, let us hear Chris's story, presented here in greater detail; he is an individual who has never admitted that he had committed sexual offences, but in all other ways, worked hard to develop a very insightful and relevant understanding of himself and his problematic behaviour. Eventually – many years after he was eligible for parole – he was released from prison, having served 12 years of an indeterminate sentence for the assault (with intent to sexually assault) and robbery of an adult woman.

Chris came over as a rather haughty and suspicious individual initially in interview, and questioned why he should talk about his personal life or matters other than his offending. With time, he mellowed in his responses, showing both a capacity for charm and a more reflective side to himself. Nevertheless, although he was quick to take responsibility for all the mistakes he had made in life, he was defensive in relation to family matters, and quick to become irritable if pressed regarding his culpability for his offending.

Chris was the youngest child in the family, having one full biological sibling – his sister – who was two years older. The children were largely brought up by their mother, as their father no longer lived with them after Chris reached the age of 4. He described his mother as a '*good mother*'; she was caring and always concerned to provide adequately for the children. Chris pointed out that without child support, his mother was often obliged to work three jobs, and would return home exhausted; although the children were sometimes minded by friendly neighbours, Chris acknowledged that he was often left to run wild after school, until his mother returned home. His sister responded well to the expectation that she should behave responsibly, taking on a few household chores and completing her homework. Her development proceeded without incident and ultimately she led a settled adult life without any obvious difficulties. Chris was quite different; he was a boisterous and active child with a rebellious streak that meant he did not like being told what to do, and rarely heeded such instructions. It is possible that at a different time and in a different family environment, he might have been thought to suffer from ADHD (attention-deficit hyperactivity disorder); who knows whether an intervention at this early stage might have shifted the direction of his pathway in life? He was disruptive at school, and often in trouble for minor scrapes in the community. With hindsight, one can see that his mother was rather erratic in her responses to him; understandably exasperated, she would sometimes punish Chris physically and impose strict curfews (that she was unable to monitor due to work commitments); at other times, she despaired and responded helplessly, simply stating tearfully that he was *'like his father'*.

At school, Chris's disruptive behaviour interfered with his academic progress; whether or not he had some specific learning difficulties was unclear, but it was certainly the case that by the time he left primary school, he was unable to read and write. The transition to secondary school is always a vulnerable time for children, and Chris was able to recount quite vividly his problems with settling into the classroom. He remembered one occasion (which stuck in my mind as a striking example), aged 11, when the children were asked to take turns in reading passages from a book out loud; he refused when it came to his turn (the reality being that he could not read, but no one knew this and he had no intention of letting himself be humiliated by revealing the deficit). When the teacher insisted he take his turn, he threw a tantrum in such a way that the teacher was forced to send him out of the classroom. This triggered the beginning of his regular truanting from school, and his reputation as a trouble-maker.

Under pressure at home and at school, Chris became more rebellious and rejecting of authority, and increasingly insistent that he be allowed to live with his estranged father – a rather romantic figure who seemed to lead an appealingly carefree and hedonistic existence. With hindsight, Chris was able to describe his father with greater clarity, as a charming but promiscuous individual who failed in his responsibilities towards various offspring, and who received Chris into his household without any expectations of discipline or adherence to rules. This was intoxicating at first, and he idolised his father as *'everything a man should be'*; he began to emulate him, and also associated increasingly with an older and highly antisocial peer group who offered excitement as part of an alternative – antisocial – code of masculine behaviour. This is sometimes referred to as delinquent identification – the development of a masculine identity based on an alternative and predominantly antisocial culture of behaviour and ideals. He acquired his first conviction for theft at the age of 14, and thereafter a series of convictions for stealing cars, robbery, and possession of cannabis and an offensive weapon (a knife).

This antisocial lifestyle included increasingly promiscuous sexual behaviour: Chris described how sexual conquests – something that came as easily to him as it had to his father – reinforced his sense of himself as a powerful and attractive personality for whom rules of fidelity and feelings of loving attachment were simply signs of weakness; he abhorred the idea of commitment and responded angrily to any sexual partner who made any claim upon him. It was within this context that Chris's first sexual conviction occurred. Aged 17, he was out *'partying'* with two friends, when they identified a girl – probably, he thought in hindsight, somewhat intoxicated – who they concluded was *'willing to party with us'*. Her witness statement clearly identified that she was out of her depth, frightened, and non-consenting, but Chris was adamant then and now that she was a willing participant. She performed oral sex on him, at his *'request'*, as she did with one of his friends, and then she left the party whilst he carried on drinking, oblivious as to the potential consequences of his behaviour. The victim went home distressed, and disclosed to her mother; police were called, Chris identified and arrested, and he subsequently received a four-year prison sentence for sexual assault.

One might imagine that for many people this highly negative outcome would trigger a good deal of reflection and a determination to change direction. However, for Chris, as an aggrieved 'victim' of a *'lying, drunken slut'* (as he described her then) and an authoritarian state, he was determined to prove that he could live on his own terms. He had managed to survive living on *'main location'* – prison wings for general prisoners, mostly avoided by convicted sex offenders for fear of attack – by strengthening his links with criminal peers and maintaining his innocence. When released back in the community, he lived mostly off illegal earnings, including dealing drugs and operating on the fringes of organised criminal activity. In other words, Chris' response to this humiliating conviction was to redouble his antisocial efforts; psychologists often describe this response as overcompensation.

The current offence – essentially an attempted rape – occurred within two years of his release. In the course of his drug-dealing activities, Chris had sometimes offered sex workers drugs in exchange for sexual favours, something that he considered at the time to be of mutual benefit. On the day of the offence, he had been particularly frustrated in response to pressure from the Job Centre, which was threatening to cut his benefits as he had made insufficient effort to find legitimate work. He felt, in retrospect, that he was angry and *'looking for a fight'*. I wondered, many years later in interview, whether the semi-public berating by a female employee had been particularly humiliating and demeaning for him (although Chris did not agree with me on this issue). Late that night he approached a woman who was clearly somewhat intoxicated and who he said he took to be a sex worker; it later transpired that she was a woman walking home from a party, drunk but not insensible, and not a sex worker. Nevertheless, as before, he offered her sex in exchange for drugs, but she refused in no uncertain terms. Enraged and in no mood to be rebuffed – *'no one says no to me and just walks on by'* – he grabbed her, stuffed a small packet of amphetamines in her pocket, and attempted to force her to perform oral sex on him; she struggled strenuously, and Chris suddenly stopped his attack – perhaps a moment of doubt? – and grabbed her handbag and ran off.

On this occasion, when convicted of an assault with intent to commit a sexual assault, Chris received a Sentence of Imprisonment for Public Protection (IPP) – a type of indeterminate sentence that was abolished in 2012, but which at the time was imposed on individuals who were thought to pose a danger to the public but whose offence did not merit a life sentence. He received a tariff (punishment period) of 7 years, and was thereafter subject to Parole Board scrutiny, eventually being released after 12 years in custody.

Chris, as already described, has maintained his denial of both the first and second sexual conviction to the present day. His progress in prison could be described as bumpy: for the first five years, he associated with other career criminals on the main wing, was suspected of dealing drugs, received adjudications (offences in breach of prison rules) for refusing orders, and generally had a reputation as a disruptive influence. Then three things happened: first, he began to realise that he would never be considered for release at his tariff point unless he was seen to be cooperating with his sentence plan; second, another prisoner that he respected helped him to learn to read and write; and third, Chris showed an aptitude for furniture restoration (a short-term workshop that had taken place in the prison), and a prison officer took an interest in him and went out of his way to source materials to support Chris's interest. Eventually, eight years into his sentence, Chris agreed to be transferred to a sex offender prison in order to complete an offending programme – despite continuing to deny that he had sexually offended.

How might we understand this change from a psychological point of view? I would suggest that initially Chris's sense of self was overly restricted to his image as an independent, macho criminal, and he was overly reliant on the views of others – namely, his father and his delinquent peer group – to sustain this restricted self-image. His sexual conviction – with all its devastating connotations of deviancy and inadequacy – meant that he had to work extra hard to maintain his self-image; denial was not sufficient in and of itself, he needed to fight the system at every opportunity. However, this is an extremely tiring position to hold year after year; with growing maturity, Chris became more aware of the need to seek alternative cognitive (or thinking) strategies, but was unable to develop a more rounded sense of self without the input of others. Becoming literate without the humiliation of exposure in the classroom was the first step to seeing himself differently; then learning a pro-social skill – identifying a talent – that did not involve rule-breaking was a second opportunity. Chris was able to identify these factors, many years later; but I would add an additional factor – the behaviour of a male prison officer intruding upon his habitual rejection of all authority figures, and challenging him to consider whether there are other ways of *'being a man'*. For these reasons, going to a sex offender prison – something that he would have strenuously resisted a few years early – posed less of a threat to his developing sense of self.

Progress, however, continued to be bumpy but in the right direction; Chris made it to open prison, but the sudden drop in security and observation levels there led to a modest resurgence in entitled behaviours – which one could describe colloquially as *'the rules don't apply to me!'* He was viewed with suspicion by staff, many of whom considered his attitude to be overly arrogant, and his choice of associates unwise. He rejected their advice, and so when it emerged that he had been bringing in a mobile phone, and had returned late from a town visit, he was sent back to closed prison. Once it was confirmed that he had not been dealing drugs with his phone but had – as he alleged – been pursuing work-related activity, it was agreed that he could return to open conditions some six months later. This was a salutary lesson for Chris who had been overly complacent about his ability to forge his own path, assuming that as long as there were no concerns of sexually inappropriate or violent behaviour, he could make his own rules.

I met with Chris before his final Parole Board hearing, when he had been returned to open prison. Without in any way presenting himself as glib or acquiescent, Chris nevertheless impressed with his grasp on *'the boy I was then'* and *'the man I want to be now'*. He spoke of his derogatory attitude towards women, his extreme selfishness and sense of entitlement, his callous behaviour towards others; he could acknowledge the pleasures of his former lifestyle – the highs, the camaraderie, the money in his pocket, the access to sex. He marked the steps evidencing change, he detailed the slow shedding of his former persona, the acquisition of a new sense of purpose and ambition. He still raged against injustice, as he perceived it, but he had found new and constructive ways to battle wrongs; his sense of grievance was short-lived rather than corrosively nurtured. In essence, he knew and accepted everything except the fact that he had committed two sexual offences.

Risk and denial

This brings us back to the central conundrum of this chapter: how can it be that an individual who denies that he has committed a sexual offence does not pose a higher risk of future sexual offending as a result of this denial? The narratives in this chapter have already enabled us to develop an understanding of denial as an avoidant strategy to manage threats to one's sense of self, to maintain self-esteem and self-image in response to shame and anxiety. To understand how this does or does not link to risk, it may be helpful to move away from the subject of sexual offending for a moment: such offences provoke such strong emotional and moral responses in all of us that it can be difficult to think clearly and objectively. Let us take an apparently irrelevant example; the story of a little boy and his mother's precious bowl….

Dan is a 5-year old boy, playing in the sitting room with some toys in a rather desultory way, while his 6-month-old baby sister is bobbing about in her rocker and contentedly waving a rattle around. Their mother is busy but keeping an eye on them until the phone rings and she is temporarily distracted as she leaves the room to chat. Dan's attention is immediately drawn to the wonderfully sparkly bowl that his mother keeps up on the shelf and which she always tells him not to touch. He clambers up on the sofa to try and touch it – he loves to feel the bobbly bits of decorative glass – and of course, he slips and knocks the bowl, which shatters on the floor. Dan is momentarily frozen with shock, he looks around but when nothing happens, he returns to his toys; peculiarly, he now seems to be utterly wrapped up in an absorbing game – the earlier incident apparently totally forgotten – when his mother returns to the room. She notes the shattered glass, and is predictably furious, her precious bowl shattered, Dan clearly having done what she had so frequently told him not to; she yells at him, in an accusatory fashion. Dan's behaviour is now rather interesting; he suddenly seems to become aware of the enormity of the situation; he looks frightened, or is it angry… some sort of mix of the two emotions, and then he does what most young children – and quite a few adults – would do, he denies it, *'it wasn't me mummy'*. Of course, he is not sufficiently sophisticated to develop a fictitious story as to how it happened, he sticks to total denial; he instinctively glances at his baby sister, almost as though he is tempted to allocate blame to her, but even at his young age, he seems to know that this is not going to be a successful strategy. He bursts into tears, and clings to his mother's legs; it's not clear whether he is trying to indicate his remorse without actually admitting guilt, or whether he is hoping to assuage her anger by presenting himself as the victim of her rage.

Dan is like any other 5 year old, and in using this example, I hope to show, yet again, how an internal feeling of guilt can be managed, but when that guilt is exposed to the view of another, denial becomes a very natural response to the shame that is evoked by such exposure. But now the question is whether Dan's denial makes him more likely to break another precious object in the future; we might add a further related question, which is whether the uncertainty regarding the sincerity of his 'remorse' also aggravates the risk of another shattered object in the future? Having stripped out the moral imperative that we feel in relation to sex offences, it is perhaps easier to understand with Dan that he is behaving normally and understandably, although immaturely. Clearly, we want him to develop a capacity to own up to misdemeanours, as this is part of the moral development necessary within a complex society. However, we can also see that his response to his mother's anger shows that he knows what he has done is wrong, and that he cares about what she thinks of him. The unpleasant feelings associated with the incident may be enough to put him off such adventures in the future – that is, we might wonder whether his desire for his mother's unconditional positive regard and the shame associated with letting her down might actually reduce the likelihood of Dan breaking objects in the future? Taking an alternative approach, what might have worried us about Dan's behaviour, in terms of future risk? Two possibilities come to mind: the first is if he had responded to his mother with callous indifference and openly admitted to breaking the vase, with a '*so what*' sort of demeanour; we know that callous and unemotional traits in young children are associated with a significantly increased risk of violence later in adolescence and early adulthood. The second concern might have been if we knew that Dan was already diagnosed with ADHD and that his lack of concentration, restlessness, and impulsive behaviour frequently got him into trouble; we might not think that bowls were specifically at risk from him, but we might think that future breakages were on the cards, and that in the short term, his mother should probably move all fragile objects well out of his reach.

Holding this example in mind, we need to return to the far more serious subject of denial and risk in those who have committed sex offences. This has been a well-studied subject, and the evidence is now unequivocal: total or partial denial in convicted sex offenders is unrelated to future risk; the research detailed in Box 3.3 provides just one robust study as an example of this evidence base. Furthermore, research also shows that when practitioners are allowed to add concerns regarding denial into their risk assessment, the accuracy of such assessments – that is, the ability to identify exactly who will go on to sexually reoffend – reduces. Finally, the research also suggests – wholly counter-intuitively – that total or partial denial in sex offenders who already pose a high risk of future sexual offending may actually be protective! That is, those high-risk men who deny are less likely to sexually reoffend than high-risk men who admit. As with Bill and our fictitious child Dan – and as we will see, with Chris as well – the factors driving denial include the ability to feel shame combined with the presence of strong attachments to others within a social network that means they care what others think about them; these are functional and protective factors.

BOX 3.3

An example of research on risk and denial

Harkins and colleagues (2014)[2] used the England and Wales Probation Service assessment system – OASys – and focused on one of the OASys questions: does the offender accept responsibility for the current offence? The researchers looked at 7,000 convicted sex offenders in relation to this question (which has a yes/no answer), and then examined their sexual reconviction rates when they were residing in the community. They found that denying responsibility was associated with a significantly *lower* sexual reoffending rate, even when they took into account the different risk levels posed by the man, as identified by a sex offender risk tool.

Chris is, of course, one of those men – a sex offender who on the basis of his history is considered to pose a high risk of sexual reoffending, and who denies his sexual offending (thereby, not taking full responsibility for all of his offending behaviours, as per the research). Although this is not primarily a chapter about risk assessment, I do need to pause for a moment and explain why it is reasonable to suggest that Chris has a high-risk history: the general sexual reconviction rate for convicted sex offenders is around 10–14%, and even though we know that not all sexual offending is identified, there is considerable evidence to suggest that the majority of sex offenders pose a fairly low risk of reoffending and that we are increasingly competent at identifying and managing risk in convicted offenders before it turns into an actual reoffence. In summary, although there is no room for complacency, it is widely accepted by experts in the field that prosecution – and all the shame and negative consequences associated with it – is in some way a deterrent to future offending in the case of sex offenders. For Chris to be high risk, there must be a number of issues or events in his history and his behaviour that differentiate him from the average; in terms of his risk profile:

1. He had a prior appearance at court for a sexual offence. Unlike most sex offenders, Chris was undeterred by his first conviction, and this raises his risk considerably.
2. He showed evidence of what we call sexual preoccupation; this is a broad term that includes the idea that sex (not simply illegal sexual aggression, but all sexual behaviour) is overly important in maintaining an individual's self-esteem and/or in regulating their mood. This might

include, in Chris's case, ideas of sexual entitlement, derogatory attitudes towards women, and a drive to enhance his image in the eyes of other men by his sexual conquests.

3. He was embroiled in an antisocial lifestyle, which is strongly associated with both sexual and violent reoffending; that is, he engaged in persistent rule-breaking, a disregard for the rights of others, he misused illegal substances, and he associated with like-minded peers who endorsed antisocial and aggressive cultural norms.

Although Chris could do nothing about his prior sexual conviction, the presence of which would always signal a heightened need for vigilance, he was able to change in relation to sexual preoccupation and antisocial lifestyle. His story indicates a process of change that was slow and characterised by setbacks, but which ultimately was evidenced by his positive response to increasing levels of freedom and responsibility. If the research suggests that Chris' denial was perhaps even protective in terms of risk, how might we understand this in practice? It seemed to me, after meeting him, that Chris had somehow created a narrative for himself that had meaning and truth within it – but which enabled him to retain his dignity. He knew as we knew that he had committed sexual offences, but by not admitting it – allowing it to remain a personal guilt rather than a public shame – he was able to construct a pathway to change that was based on ideas of redemption rather than condemnation.

A redemptive narrative is not the same as a truthful narrative, and this is something that is challenging for practitioners – and the public – to accept as meaningful and valid. Yet we know from theories of desistance – a compelling criminological approach to understanding how repeat offenders eventually give up offending behaviour – that redemptive narratives are one of the key mechanisms by which desistance is achieved. Chris' story is one that exemplifies the central role that a person's sense of self needs to take in their pathway to change.

Notes

1. https://ccrc.gov.uk/case-library/ https://www.innocenceproject.org/all-cases/#sex-crimes
2. Harkins, L., Howard, P., Barnett, G., Wakeling, H., & Miles, C. (2014). Relationships between denial, risk and recidivism in sexual offenders. *Archives Sexual Behavior*, *44*, 157–166.

Further reading

I have two recommendations for understanding the issues of denial and sex offending more clearly. The first provides a reasonably up-to-date overview of the relevant research findings in relation to denial and risk:

Craissati, J. (2015). Should we worry about sex offenders who deny their offences? *Probation Journal: The Journal of Community and Criminal Justice*, 1–11.

The second recommendation on denial is a book that is rather out-of-date now, but has two excellent chapters on understanding denial and intervening using motivational interviewing techniques:

Erooga, M., Morrison, T., & Beckett, R. (1994). *Sexual Offending Against Children: Assessment and Treatment of Male Abusers*. Routledge. Chapters 3 and 4, pp. 55–101.

There are numerous publications on the risk assessment of sex offenders, but a good starting point would be:

Craissati, J. (2004). *Managing High Risk Sex Offenders in the Community: A Psychological Approach*. Routledge.

There are also numerous websites that provide access to more academic and specialist risk-related information. An informative American site is SMART, the Office of Sex Offender Sentencing, Monitoring, Apprehending, Registering, and Tracking (https://www.smart.gov/SOMAPI/sec1/ch6_risk.html). In Canada, risk assessment work undertaken by the government is presented on the Static 99 website (static99.org). Some more general guidance on risk assessment in England and Wales can be found in the *National Offender Management Service Public Protection Manual*, 16th edition. https://www.justice.gov.uk/downloads/offenders/psipso/psi-2016/psi-18-2016-pi-17-2016-public-protection-manual.pdf.

Finally, for further information on desistance theory, a good starting point might be:

Maruna, S. (2001). *Making Good: How Ex-Convicts Reform and Rebuild Their Lives*. Washington, DC: American Psychological Association Books.

For those with sexual convictions specifically, I would recommend:

Laws, R., & Ward, T. (2010). *Desistance from Sex Offending: Alternatives to Throwing Away the Keys*. New York: The Guilford Press.

David and Eddie's story 4

Understanding the impact of a childhood in care in relation to later violent offending

David and Eddie's story

David and Eddie both were in their 20s when they were convicted – in separate incidents – of Section 18 Wounding, and each received a custodial sentence of ten years. Section 18 Wounding – also referred to as Section 18 Grievous Bodily Harm (GBH) which is very similar – is a seriously violent offence in which significant bodily harm (physical or psychological) is caused to the victim; the harm has to be intended and caused 'unlawfully and maliciously'; that is, it cannot be understood as an act of self-defence, or relate to harm that was unintended.

David and Eddie both had been 'looked after' children, having spent time in local authority care (see Box 4.1 for a definition), but their experiences of care and how it influenced their pathway into violent crime were very different. This chapter is about that pathway, exploring the way in which experiences of state-appointed parental authority can adversely influence the choices and decisions made by individuals who end up serving long prison sentences for serious crimes. It builds on an understanding of attachment and developmental adversity that was first introduced in Chapter 2 in relation to Adam's story.

BOX 4.1

A definition for being in care

Children who are in care are referred to as 'looked after'. Under the Children Act (1989), a child is legally defined as 'looked after' by a local authority if s/he is provided with accommodation for a continuous period for more than 24 hours, and is subject to a care order or a placement order. A child ceases to be 'looked after' at the age of 18.

The care system as a matter of social concern

It may seem self-evident that time in a care as a child adversely affects one's life chances: inadequate parenting, disrupted schooling, poorly paid staff who are overworked and undervalued, negative peer influences, and so on are all likely to play a part. Nevertheless, it seems to me that the scale of the problem – as a social rather than psychological issue – requires some elaboration and emphasis. Box 4.2 provides a few statistics to demonstrate why we should be concerned about the outcome of a child's contact with the care system, and most particularly, how children are criminalised as a result of being 'looked after'.

The statistics speak for themselves. The National Audit Office (2016), the Howard League for Penal Reform (2016), and the Prison Reform Trust (2016)[1] all raised concerns regarding the criminalisation of children in care. The reports identified the low threshold for foster carers – and most particularly for staff in children's homes – for reporting a child's misdemeanours to the police (tolerating challenging behaviour much less than the average parent); and how children who went missing were more likely to be remanded to an institution when apprehended by the police. I would suggest that the elevated misuse of substances by looked after adolescents that is highlighted in the statistics is a driver for offences of theft – to fund substance misuse – and this in turn is likely to raise the likelihood of repeated appearances in court incurring increasingly harsh penalties for the teenagers.

What then happens to these children as they transition into adulthood? There seems to be little or no information on the types of crime that individuals commit who have a history of having been placed in care. What we do know is that there are fairly consistent findings to suggest that around 25% of all prisoners have been in care at some point as a child, and that 7% of all prisoners have spent most of their childhood in care; clearly, this is disproportionately high as compared to the 1% or so of the general population

BOX 4.2

'Looked after' children: why we should be concerned

Some statistics

- About 1% of the general population has been in care as a child; currently 75,000 children are 'looked after', of whom around 90% are in foster care and around 10% are in institutions or children's homes.
- Around 60% of 'looked after' children have emotional, behavioural, and educational difficulties. Approximately 50% have substance misuse problems that require intervention.
- Only 12% of children who have been in care achieve five A*–C grade GCSEs compared to 52% of children who have not been in care. When leaving care at the age of 18, 41% of 18 year olds have no involvement in training, education, or employment as compared to 15% of the general 18-year-old population.
- About 1% of the general population has a criminal conviction. For those who were in care as a child, about 5–6% had acquired a criminal conviction.
- For those children who were placed in institutions (such as secure residential provision and children's homes) rather than foster care, 19% had acquired a criminal conviction by the age of 15. That is, they were 20 times more likely to have a criminal conviction than a child who has not been in care.
- Around 50% of convicted children in custody (for example, Young Offender Institutions) have been in care.

who has been in care as a child. There seems to be some additional evidence that prisoners who have been in care as a child are more likely to service short-term sentences (suggesting that they have committed less serious crimes or non-violent crimes – quite possibly, offences related to theft as discussed above), but they are more likely to be reconvicted than those prisoners without a care history.

Shocking as these statistics are, it is important to remember that for most children who are 'looked after' – particularly those who are in care for less than 12 months and who have had a stable foster placement – the outcomes are largely positive. Most return to their parents in a timely manner, and do not offend and are not criminalised; many go on to higher education and work in early adulthood. There are numerous ways in which individuals are resilient, in terms of their personal characteristics, their early attachment experiences, and their opportunities in life.

Making sense of the psychological impact of the care system on an individual's pathway to violence

Statistics make a point, but do not resonate at the individual level. Statistics are not nuanced, and cannot help us understand the individual narratives involved. David and Eddie may have acquired identical convictions at similar ages, and both been in care, but their narratives that make sense of these experiences are very different. We meet them as they are recently released from prison, and are resident in an Approved Premises – the name for hostels staffed 24/7 and managed by the probation service – where more serious offenders are required to reside for a few months after leaving prison and before moving on to independent accommodation. We can see that their life trajectories seem to be rather different: David has used his time in prison constructively, and is successful in his second parole application – he was allowed to apply for parole at the mid-point in his sentence – and was released after six years in prison, with the proviso that he would be directly supervised by the probation service for a further two years or so, and thereafter would be required to be of 'good behaviour' for the final part of his ten-year sentence. Any breach of his licence requirements during this time in the community could result in his return to prison. Eddie, serving exactly the same sentence as David, is released automatically at the two-thirds point in his sentence, although he remains in prison for a few extra months as he was serving extra time for bad behaviour. He had a much more turbulent prison record than David, and had considered it not worth his time applying for parole. Out after seven years in prison, Eddie has only one year under the direct supervision of the probation service, but otherwise is managed in the same way as David.

David's story

David had attracted some negative attention during his first few weeks in the Approved Premises; staff found him rather cold and aloof, and he was prone to pointing out and asserting his rights if he felt staff were being inconsistent or withholding. But he was an intelligent person who clearly understood where the limits lay. I noticed in my first meeting with him that there was no question of earning his respect or his trust with any simple strategies: careful listening and empathic responses were not enough to convince him that I had anything of significant value to offer.

David was the youngest child of four, and the only one who later got into trouble at school and with the police; his two sisters were settled with families, and his brother settled down after a slightly rebellious period in adolescence, and had steady employment. David acknowledged that he was rather a spoilt child as the baby of the family; he adored his father who was quite often absent from the family home, but when there, made his presence felt. He was an imposing physical presence, and David could recall being lifted onto his father's knee and being 'shown off' to visiting relatives. Although very hazy about his father's activities at the time, David later learnt that he was a career criminal – someone who made a living from quite sophisticated and organised acquisitive crime such as armed robberies – and his periods of absence were related to going into hiding, interspersed with short prison sentences. His father imparted a strong – albeit somewhat criminal – moral code, which David remembered as him being encouraged to stand up for himself physically in response to perceived injustice, never to '*thieve off your own*', and never to hit a woman. David's relationship with his mother was less close, although she was a dutiful mother and made sure that he was adequately clothed, fed, and disciplined. She was closer to and more affectionate with her daughters, and David was aware of a slight sense that his mother held his father in some contempt, and this attitude spilled over towards him. She was, for example, particularly strict towards him if he was mischievous, and was very quick to counteract his father's pride in him if he was rebellious or won a fight at primary school. She often disciplined him with a slipper and grounded him in his room for weeks at a time; he reflected that it sometimes felt like she was trying to '*beat my father out of me*', and he became resentful of what he perceived to be her '*unfair attitude*'.

At the age of 10, David's parents separated; this followed a period of time of growing arguments between them, although there was never any physical violence. Piecing together events in hindsight, David realised that the final blow to the marriage was his father's arrest for armed robbery; the couple divorced shortly after his father received a 16-year prison sentence, and David never saw him again as there was no question of his mother allowing him to visit his father in prison; his father died ten years later whilst David was serving his current sentence. David's mother kept the family together by dint of hard work. However, her relationship with him deteriorated during the following 12 months; she was tired, irritable, and increasingly ferocious in her attempts to control him. He resented his mother, blamed her for his father's absence, and became increasingly rebellious both at home and at school. It is unfortunate that this difficult year coincided with David's transition to secondary school, a vulnerable time for all children as they learn to acclimatise to a more exacting school regime and the temptations of a more diverse peer group with greater levels of freedom out of school. His mother was at the end of her tether, her limited capacity to tolerate his defiance exhausted, and she voluntarily liaised with the local authority to have him placed into care as a result of him being behaviourally out of her control.

David eloquently described his transition into the care system, and his transformation from a mischievous, overconfident, and rather entitled child into a callously indifferent delinquent. The first shock to which he had to acclimatise was his relocation from a rather sleepy suburb to a deprived inner city location; this was via a few months in a foster family placement that broke down because David was still a very angry boy who was not yet prepared to accept any authority except his father's. Back again in the children's home, with one failed placement behind him, it seemed that no one held out much hope of another foster placement succeeding; and David compounded this belief by insisting that he would stay in the children's home. Many years later in the Approved Premises, David still remembered the staff in the home with contempt, resisting any attempts by others to suggest a more balanced perspective on the predicament of the staff's situation. His experience was held at a deeply emotional level, and had scarred him: he experienced the staff as ineffective with and/or indifferent to the children, a 'travesty' of their role as carers. He described how they struggled to control the children, and so resorted to threatening and bullying tactics, often using humiliation as a means of control. He himself was referred to as 'weak' when staff told other children that he had wet the bed when he first arrived; he was beaten in front of others for fighting in the bedroom, and beaten again when he ran off from the home. Punishments were inflicted indiscriminately and so were experienced by him as excessive and unfair; treats were occasionally available – for example, a trip to the skating rink – but seemed to be allocated according to favourites, and so were not worth striving for. David, already an angry boy, became a furiously angry teenager.

Delinquent identification was a phrase introduced in Chapter 3 (page 30). In David's case, his strong attachment to his father – incorporating his father's criminal code of conduct – was reflected in his identification with the older delinquent peers at the children's home. He sought their approval, as he might once have sought his father's approval, and in them he found a connection or relationship that seemed to be predictable and consistent, with rules of engagement that he understood as logical and fair. As their gofer, he was constantly operating on the fringes of illegal activity; however, his first formal criminal act was when he broke into a locker at school with a couple of friends, and found some cannabis that he went on to sell. With the proceeds, he bought a new pair of trainers, and – as he put it later – his fate was sealed. He could recall the memory of that moment as though it were yesterday: the excitement of the break in, the thrill of the discovery, the ease with which he could make money, and the immense satisfaction of owning a desirable object that raised his value in the eyes of others. By the age of 15, David acquired his first criminal conviction; thereafter, as a rather bright young man, he managed to evade police attention for some of the time, but the development of a problematic crack cocaine habit meant that his offending behaviour became increasingly impulsive. Operating with peers, he was caught for a number of street robberies, and was found to be in possession of an offensive weapon on one occasion. David admitted that carrying a weapon was habitual for him in late adolescence / early adulthood; his weapon of choice was a small cosh, as knives were *'for suckers'* (because, as he explained it, knives were more likely to result in an unintended fatal outcome). David adhered to a firm view of himself as a non-violent criminal with a strong moral code: yes, he could be verbally threatening and he used his physical presence in a deliberately intimidating manner, but he believed that he was in control of all the criminal situations in which he found himself, and could direct the outcome, without recourse to violence, rather as though he were a director on a film set.

The offence of Wounding (with intent to cause Grievous Bodily Harm, Section 18) took place within this context. David, and two associates, intended to carry out the robbery of a small jewellery store manager as he walked down the street with the day's takings in his secure briefcase. Their preparation for the robbery had been somewhat cursory – they had been given the information by a third party and knew the route that the store manager would take to the safety deposit box. Their thinking had undoubtedly been negatively influenced by their drug habit, and David described himself, in hindsight, as craving another hit of crack cocaine at the time, and therefore his thinking was clouded, he was irritable and impulsively determined to pursue the robbery. On the day, he saw the jewellery manager leave the shop, and chased after him, grabbing the case; however, the victim had a very firm grip on the case, and swung his arm – and the case – in an attempt to push David away and extricate himself from the situation. David stumbled and the victim ran off; he said that at that point, he was so startled by the victim's unexpected response that his heart started racing and he began to feel that he was in a dream-like sequence in which time slowed down. Without a clear thought in his head, he chased after the victim once again and was unaware that he had pulled out his cosh from his back pocket. Grabbing the victim once more, David made no attempt to grab the case again, but started to bludgeon him with the cosh; the victim quickly fell to the ground, but David felt unable to stop at that point, and continued to hit him repeatedly. It was only when he saw the blood pouring out from a head wound that he had inflicted that David seemed to come to

BOX 4.3

Instrumental or reactive aggression?

Instrumental aggression refers to a behaviour – aggressive or violent – intended to achieve a goal. It is likely to be proactive, premeditated, or intentional. The goal might be external (money from an armed robbery) or internal (wanting control over someone). It may be vengeful, but the anger will be 'cold' and the retaliation planned.

Reactive aggression (sometimes called expressive or hostile) refers to aggressive or violent behaviour stemming from a feeling of anger – often triggered by a perceived threat – which induces a feeling of fear. Such threats usually include the anticipation of humiliation or rejection by others. The aggression is impulsive in nature and self-preservative; that is, hitting out at the source of the threat in order to defend oneself.

his senses; he stopped, looked around him, and then ran off (without the case). He was quickly identified and caught by the police.

Pausing for a moment in the narrative, it may be that there are readers who are sceptical about aspects of David's account of the offence itself – despite being factually corroborated by what the victim could recall of events. It may be helpful to highlight two rather technical psychological issues that require clarification. First, David describes a state of *dissociation* that is commonly described by individuals who commit violent offences associated with very intense levels of emotion, such as rage or fear. Dissociation is the word used to describe a state of detachment or disconnection from immediate physical and emotional experiences; individuals often describe a trance-like state, a sense of time slowing, being in a film, or watching themselves. It's not dissimilar to the stories that athletes tell about serious injuries of which they were entirely unaware in the moment they occurred; pain that is only experienced when the adrenaline drive has subsided.

The second technical element of the offence story is the shift from what we call *instrumental aggression* (the use of threat to control the behaviour of the recipient in order that we can achieve our aim) to *reactive aggression* (the use of violence to express intense emotions relating to anger or panic). It is worryingly common that individuals, whose sole intention is to steal, are prone to responding excessively violently when the victim does not behave as expected. For example, there are sometimes newspaper reports of female victims of street robberies who do not let go of their handbag and are dragged into the path of a car or beaten; burglaries can result in violence when the victim unexpectedly appears in the house, inadvertently blocking the burglar's exit. Studies of the use of weapons in acquisitive crimes support this idea of the potential for instrumental aggression to turn into reactive aggression when adrenaline surges and the victim does not behave in the expected manner.

Returning to David, we can see from his story that although his experiences in care in no way predetermined the outcome – such a brutally violent offence – they shaped a series of choices that he made subsequently. The seeds were sown in his early attachments, the way in which he learnt to think about himself as male, modelling himself on his indulgent but criminal father, his anger in response to unfairness, and his preoccupation with a moral code that was rational and predictable. Being in care at a pivotal point in his development then nurtured these problematic shoots and provided him with opportunities to replicate his idealised relationship with his father, and to follow in his footsteps; it developed into a view of authority as fundamentally duplicitous and reinforced his insistence that he would only submit to the authority of those he respected.

Eddie's story

Eddie was quite a character; he had a quick witted and charmingly childlike quality that tended to evoke a rather maternal response in staff; that is, until he tested positive for cocaine two weeks after his release, lost his temper with the hostel manager when given a written warning as a result, and startled staff with the ferocity of his subsequent verbal attack. Yet within minutes it was as if the incident had never occurred and he went off quite happily, discussing the latest events in one of the TV soap operas with his keyworker. Although willing to meet with me, he was lacking curiosity about the purpose of the interview, and was a rather challenging interviewee in terms of his distractibility – fiddling with objects in the room and pausing to listen whenever there were noises outside the room – and his incoherence. The latter point was particularly striking in terms of his difficulty in providing an account of his life that had any consistent sequencing or coherence; he jumped from event to event in a random order, and confidently insisted on details that were clearly contradicted by the documentation I had available. There seemed to be two narrative plots to his life: the first was one that had been put together by various professionals, each drawing on the material available; seen from the perspective of the professional, Eddie's life story was a depressing tale of neglect and deprivation. The second narrative plot was the one that Eddie had written for himself which coincided with the professionals' narrative here and there, but was altogether more dramatic and compelling, a story of the little person standing up to authority, a tale of thwarted love.

Eddie was 4 years old when he and his younger brother were taken into care. Reports are rather sparse, but state that his mother was a drug addict and sex worker who grossly neglected the children in terms of basic care and affection, and who exposed them to frightening scenes of violence in the home when she brought clients back or when her pimp beat her up. Eddie's account is that his mother was the victim of both sexual and physical violence; she was raped by her father repeatedly, and he himself was the product of another rape incident, the perpetrator being unknown to him. The children were rescued by the local authority when his mother was away – for unclear reasons – for a period of several days. After a few months in a children's home, both boys were placed with an experienced foster family; Eddie's younger brother was adopted within a year, but Eddie was a wild and rather uncontrollable boy with a terrible temper, some learning difficulties, and an intense loyalty towards his mother which meant that he was rejecting all attempts to forge a substitute attachment with him. He never forgave his brother for agreeing to be adopted, and rejected all subsequent offers of contact with him. His foster family went to great efforts to bond with him, but after a further year or so, the placement broke down; the family's biological son was about to sit his GCSEs and the parents were concerned to protect him from all the additional stress of Eddie's behaviour during this important time in his life. By the age of 8, Eddie was back in a children's home, and there he stayed.

Eddie's view was that his foster carers had been quite kind, but really their motive was about the money that came with fostering. He had always felt sure that his mother would come to fetch him back home, but he realised that the authorities were hostile to her, and he believed – possibly correctly – that they had hidden his whereabouts from her. He said that he chanced upon his mother in the street one day – he was aged about 10 – and instantly recognised her. She said that she had been searching for him everywhere, and they exchanged phone numbers, with his mother promising to *'get him out of the home just as soon as I can get my life together'*. He tried to ring her two days later, but her number was no longer available; nevertheless, he was convinced of her sincere intentions and felt that the following few years were largely about *'waiting for her at weekends, expecting her to turn up'*. Eddie described the children's home as *'the good life'*: he was clearly out of the control of the staff and seemed to have considerable freedom; he told endless anecdotes of climbing out of windows at night to roam the streets, the camaraderie he forged with his peers, *'bunking off school'* (truanting), and smoking stolen packets of cigarettes in the park. The twinkle in his eye only dimmed when he returned to the *'useless bunch of idiots'* (the staff) and the malicious intent of the social workers in preventing him and his mother being reunited.

By the age of 12, Eddie had his first criminal conviction for theft; this was quickly followed by a series of convictions for criminal damage (destroying property), burglaries (from building sites), and then progressing to street robberies. Although Eddie referred to his *'mates'*, in actual fact the majority of his offences were committed alone; I speculated that he was probably too much of a liability for the other children in the home, too volatile, too unpredictable, too reckless for them. He was known for his hair trigger temper, and this was most apparent when approached by authority; as he acquired a reputation locally, it was often the police who bore the brunt of his aggression; taunting them became a compelling game for him, and by the age of 15 he acquired his first conviction for assault and found himself in a Borstal (a type of youth detention centre intended to reform youth). For several years, a depressingly inevitable cycle occurred: substance misuse, thieving to fund his drug habit, provoking and assaulting the police when arrested, incarceration in a Young Offenders Institution (a type of prison for adolescents and young adults), extra time for hitting prison staff, release and renewed substance misuse. By this time, Eddie was habitually carrying a weapon – a knife – having himself been stabbed on a previous occasion. It never occurred to him that anything other than going out *'tooled up'* was the norm.

It was within this context that the current offence of Wounding with intent took place. Eddie had recently been released from prison, he was using drugs again and he was homeless. He openly acknowledged that he was after cash, and had previously stolen from the newsagent where he now headed. The shop was empty except for the owner behind the counter; Eddie pulled out his knife and ordered him to open the till. Then without any provocation, Eddie suddenly started screaming at the shop owner, incoherent words mostly, but the victim's witness statement identified the following: *'what the f*** are you looking at... you taking the piss?'* from Eddie. Eddie's account was that he was high, having taken crack cocaine earlier that morning; the victim infuriated him with a glance that seemed to be sneering at him. He agreed that he viewed the victim as *'taking the piss'*, and admitted his subsequent violence, which he now viewed as excessive, although he had *'been provoked'*. Eddie grabbed the victim's hair and slammed his head down on the counter, before taking his knife and slashing him across his face.

Eddie's prison sentence had been rather turbulent, characterised by numerous assaults on prison officers as soon as he perceived them to be either unfair in exerting their authority, or applying the rules with insufficient respect. With female staff he was more reflective and, as described above, more likely to evoke a rather maternal and caring response from them. His excellent female probation officer had forged quite a good working relationship with him, although she made an interesting remark, when we discussed the case – that he was 'as slippery as an eel.... [T]here's something that's just skin deep about him' – which I found to be insightful but worrying.

Epilogue

It will come as no surprise to learn that David and Eddie had different outcomes on this occasion. David completed his time on probation licence, and successfully completed his time to the end of sentence. His pathway to a non-offending lifestyle was not without a few bumps – for example, receiving a police caution for verbal abuse after being rather brusquely challenged by a policeman on his way home after an evening drinking in the pub – but essentially he had the motivation and the ability to 'make good'. The pathway to desisting from crime is as meandering as the pathway into crime: for David, he was able to seek out an intimate relationship with a woman who came from a deprived but essentially pro-social family, and his interpersonal skills and capacity for intimacy were good enough for him to be able to sustain this relationship, and to seek out and connect to a wider social network. Eventually, he also obtained legitimate employment with a friend of his brother's, after a difficult period of multiple rejections by employers advertising with the Job Centre. Work and relationship were central to consolidating his sense of himself as a capable provider; with the birth of his first child, he began to mellow, and allowed himself to experience tender and protective feelings. By the time I lost touch with David's progress, some years later, the longer term outcome was looking good. Nevertheless, I anticipated that there might be some challenges ahead with family life: David was prone to a fairly black and white style of thinking and I wondered whether his approach to parenting might perhaps be overly rigid. I also thought that there may be some difficulties in his relationship along the line, with him being overly controlling; but I took some comfort from the probation officer's account of David's partner as a sensible and assertive young woman, protective of her child and independently minded.

Eddie, on the other hand, was recalled to prison within a couple of weeks of our meeting at the probation hostel: he had persisted in his substance misuse following release – receiving positive drug test results – and was eventually suspected of stealing from other more vulnerable residents at the hostel. He seemed to be impervious to the efforts of the hostel staff to manage him with either discipline or care; he was a chameleon whose demeanour bore no resemblance to his behaviour. Once back in prison, he was hugely disruptive and assaultive, ensuring that he was rapidly placed in the segregation unit in prison, and then subject to repeated transfers from prison to prison. No one seemed able to forge a meaningful relationship with him – his behaviour ensuring that there was no opportunity to do this – and he was destined to serve the remainder of his sentence in custody. It is perhaps telling that I was unable to find out what happened to Eddie after his eventual release at the end of sentence; it was no surprise that he seemed to be invisible – the real story of his life – never held in mind, and making no impression unless he was a nuisance. This recalled to mind something another individual had once said to me (someone with greater insight and capacity to reflect): he said *'how can I stop fighting the system? When I cause trouble, I get a response and I know I exist; if I stopped, then I would be nothing'*. I felt outlook for Eddie was depressingly bleak; there seemed to be little indication of maturation or the mellowing of destructive behaviours that usually occur with ageing. It was certainly too soon to write him off, but I wondered whether he was destined to follow the pathway of endless revolving door returns to prison, to the point where he became so accustomed to institutional life that he would never be able to function in the community; it was either that or the possibility of early death from a drug overdose, impetuous behaviour, or at the hands of his violent peers.

David and Eddie are not necessarily representative of the wider group of individuals in prison who had have experiences in care as a child; but the focus in this book is on seriously violent individuals, not those who steal. Even though Eddie's story, in particular, is extreme, the contrast between David and Eddie is instructive. With the benefit of hindsight, we can see that the stability in David's early life became more clearly influential in determining his capacity to desist from crime as he approached his 30s; although not without its problems, his childhood was characterised by affection and fairly consistent nurturing, and he had access to moral and social codes or ways of life that provided structure to the way in which he interacted with others. Being placed into care at a time when he was angry, and embarking on the usual task of adolescence – developing a sense of himself as man, separate from his family and seeking attachments to his peers and to social institutions – led to a period of problematic behaviour that required time and reflection to resolve. Nevertheless, the 'good enough' foundations of his early development were able to emerge as he matured; furthermore, his intelligence and his resolve – despite being anti-authoritarian and challenging at times – were additional protective factors.

For Eddie, the fundamental building bricks of secure attachment leading to a consistent and coherent sense of himself in relation to others were entirely missing from his impoverished early childhood. It was as though he had shaped an alternative narrative for himself that masked the emptiness of his emotional life and his inability to forge a meaningful connection to others. I would speculate that facing this fundamental absence within himself was too devastating for him, and so he deployed all his energies in maintaining the mask and avoiding connection to others. His likeability – particularly his ability to evoke a maternal response in female practitioners – was a protective factor, but his drive to keep all those with 'parental authority' at bay overwhelmed both him and those who wanted to help him. For Eddie, life in care provided a solution that we might find intolerable to contemplate, but which for him facilitated the preservation of a precarious sense of himself.

Note

1. National Audit Office (2016). Children in Need of Help or Protection. Department for Education.
   Howard League for Penal Reform (2016). Criminal Care. London: The Howard League for Penal Reform
   Prison Reform Trust (2016). In Care. Out of Trouble.

Frank's story 5

Understanding how sexual victimisation in childhood might be linked to the abuse of others in adulthood

The focus of this chapter is on the victim to abuser pathway, specifically exploring the way in which an experience of sexual victimisation in childhood might be linked to becoming a perpetrator of a sexual offence in adulthood. Later in this chapter, Frank's detailed narrative brings this pathway to life, particularly in terms of how we unravelled the impact of his trauma on him through the course of our therapeutic relationship, as well as understanding how it linked to his subsequent offending. However, in the first instance, I need to lay out some facts about the victim to abuser pathway, and in particular, elaborate on the ways in which men with sexual convictions talk about their childhood sexual victimisation and how it affected them. Frank's sexual offences were against children, but this chapter is about all those with sexual convictions, including those with adult victims.

Victim to perpetrator: a few facts

As is always the case in this book, my focus remains on those who offend, and therefore the huge body of evidence that responds to the wider question of childhood sexual abuse and its impact on victims who do not become perpetrators is not touched upon here. There is, however, a much smaller body of evidence that explores:

- Whether or not being sexually abused as a child increases the likelihood of becoming a perpetrator of child sexual abuse (or all sexual offences) in adulthood?
- What are the characteristics of sexually abused boys who may be at greater risk of becoming a perpetrator in adulthood?

Box 5.1 outlines the limited number of key facts that are reasonably well established. The figures provide a really nice example of how statistics can be quoted to suit our purposes, potentially painting a misleading picture. The truthful answer to the question 'does being sexually abused as a child raise your chances of becoming a sexual offender as an adult?' is yes. However, the truthful answer to the question 'does being sexually abused as a child make you likely to become a sexual offender as an adult?' is no. As can be seen from Box 5.1, although victimisation leads to a ten-fold increase in likelihood, it is only a small minority of boys who become perpetrators as an adult. Similarly, although men with sexual convictions report very high levels of sexual victimisation as a child, at least half such individuals – if not more – have not had childhood sexual victimisation experiences. What should we conclude from this? Being sexually abused as

BOX 5.1

Victim to perpetrator statistics

1. Approximately **1%** of the male population in England and Wales acquires a sexual conviction over the course of their lifetime.

   \+

   Around **10%** of boys who have been sexually abused as a child go on to acquire a sexual conviction as an adult.

   =

   Being sexually abused as a child makes boys *ten* times more likely to become a perpetrator in adulthood *but* **90%** of sexually abused boys don't become perpetrators.
2. Somewhere around **30–50%** of men with sexual convictions against children have been sexually abused as a child. This is much higher in those men who have male victims (around **80–90%**).

   Somewhere around **20–30%** of men with sexual convictions against adult women have been sexually abused as a child.

   These figures compare with an estimated **5–10%** of the general male population who have been sexually abused as children.

a child is highly relevant to understanding the pathway to sexual offending later in adulthood, but it is not the whole story by any means.

There is only a small amount of research that seeks to identify what the characteristics of these vulnerable boys might be (probably because studies are methodologically complex and potentially unethical to conduct): these prospective studies (that is, following up children to see what happens to them) suggest that the boys most vulnerable to becoming perpetrators having been sexually abused as children are those who live within emotionally neglectful and possibly physically abusive families. That is, there are additional features of their early family life – including attachment issues as we discussed in Chapter 2 – that are necessarily present before the risk of a pathway to sexual offending develops. If we look at retrospective studies (that is, ask offending adults about their childhood experiences), then a few more characteristics emerge. Such sexually abused perpetrators are more likely than non-abused perpetrators:

- To have come from emotionally abusive and neglectful families, particularly if, as adults, they pose a higher risk to others.
- To have engaged in 'sex play' with other boys of their age, when they were children.
- Never to have attempted to disclose their abuse until they were sentenced for their adult sexual conviction. Or,
- To have disclosed the offence as a child, but for this to have resulted in being beaten or reabused by the person to whom they disclosed the abuse.
- To have diverse sexual interests as an adult.
- To be uncertain or anxious as to their sexual orientation as an adult.

Stories about the disclosure and impact of sexual victimisation as a child

Group treatment approaches for men with sexual convictions have changed and developed in line with research over the years, but at any one point in time, most groups are fairly similar to each other; considering sexual victimisation tends to form a fairly small part of any such treatment approach. Nevertheless, the experience of talking about victimisation experiences within a group of male perpetrators, many of whom prefer to emphasise their strengths rather than contemplate their vulnerabilities, can be influential in changing everyone's thinking. The following extracts provide snapshots from group members reflecting on their childhood experiences in a programme where 50% of group members had been sexually abused, none of whom had successfully disclosed their abuse as children. These very brief vignettes illustrate their reflections with other group members:

Gary Gary was struggling in the group programme as a rather hostile and resistant member. He insisted on describing his offence as *'a relationship'* even though the victim was an 8-year-old boy and he was in his 30s. He had always maintained that he was raped, aged 15, when leaving a night club that he should not have been attending; he said that he told his mother, the police were called, but the perpetrator never apprehended. After six months in the group, when completing a related group task, he broke down and confessed that he had made up this incident; *'the truth is, that I was sexually abused, but it was by a neighbour who used to give me money and sweets to let him touch me. … [I]t went on and on, at least a year and I kept going back quite willingly, I just wanted the stuff he gave me. … I don't know why I kept going'*. He never disclosed the abuse, largely because he felt he was complicit with what happened, and he blamed himself entirely. The group members managed to be very mature and supportive in their response to Gary, and their insistence that he was not to blame seemed to represent a turning point for him in the group.

Comments Sometimes sexually abused boys feel primarily a sense of personal guilt for what occurred, having apparently consented at a superficial level, given the lack of overt physical coercion involved in some of the experiences. This was particularly noticeable with Gary who felt the need to invent a violent stranger attack in order to mask his shame about his actual experiences as a child.

Harry Harry was sexually abused by a teacher at school on two occasions over one month when he was about 12. He told his mother, but she beat him ferociously when she heard his story, calling him a *'dirty, lying bastard'*, and nothing further was said about it. When discussing his offences against his stepdaughter about 30 years later – at a time when he was aggrieved with his wife for going out to work in a pub every evening – he said *'I can't really tell you why I did it, but now I think there was something about me being angry, but angry all out* *of proportion to the situation.... I wanted to get back at my wife, I thought I could spoil something (her daughter) that she cared about.... I wanted her to take me seriously*'. Later Harry began to be able to make some links between these two experiences – as victim not only of his abuser but of his mother, and how this then related to him as perpetrator.

Comments An important ingredient that seems to fuel the victim to perpetrator pathway is the experience of abuse occurring within an emotionally barren or problematic family context – such as for Harry – in which not only can these difficult victim experiences not be safely shared, but where disclosure elicits a personal attack from those who should protect.

Ian Ian was groomed by a man whom he met online over a period of a year, eventually meeting up with him and embarking on a number of sexual encounters with this individual as well as a number of his acquaintances that he introduced to Ian. This took place during Ian's adolescence, and he told no one largely because he worried that he must be homosexual in orientation since he had willingly met these men and had been sexually aroused during their sexual contact. His anxiety was all the more acute since he was insistent that it '*would be wrong to be gay*', a belief that mirrored his father's attitude. Although he was very shy with girls his own age, in his mid-20s he had his first girlfriend – a young woman of 18 with mild learning difficulties. In the group programme, Ian was able to recognise that his girlfriend's vulnerability was important because he felt less threatened by her than by other women to whom he had been attracted. He and his girlfriend had had a sexual relationship which initially appeared to be consenting; however, as his girlfriend began to distance herself from him – she felt stifled by his neediness and possessiveness towards her – he became more sexually aggressive towards her, until eventually he raped her on at least one occasion. Later in the group programme, Ian was able to identify how his anxieties about being homosexual had led him to the situation in which '*I needed sex with **** to reassure myself that I wasn't gay; if she said no, I felt panicky ... angry... kind of frantic really.*'

Comments Ian struggled with questions about 'why me' that transformed into anxieties about his masculinity and his sexual orientation – *'am I weak, am I abnormal, am I homosexual?'* For a boy particularly, his sexual arousal is highly noticeable to himself as well as to others in terms of his erection, and seems to indicate that he is a willing and aroused participant in a sexual act that he may in fact experience as abhorrent or frightening at an emotional level (even though he responds differently at a physical level).

John John never agreed that he was sexually abused as a child, and more generally, resisted any idea that he had suffered from adversity or neglect when young; any suggestion of vulnerability was received by him as offensive and demeaning. Nevertheless, when the group was talking about early sexual experiences, it emerged that he had had a sexual relationship for six months with his best friend's mother (he was 14, she was in her mid-30s). His perspective was that *'I would have been the envy of all my mates if they'd known.... [L]earning from an experienced woman ... super cool, she made me so confident, I knew I could have any girl I wanted after that'*. In reality, none of his friends knew about it as the woman had insisted they keep it a secret to avoid envious criticism – *'we knew no one would understand it was special'*. He was adamant that his later rape conviction – sexually assaulting a woman that he picked up in a night club and who had rebuffed his advances in front of his mates – was unconnected to this early experience. This may well have been the case, although the group leaders felt that his sexual victimisation – make no mistake, that is what it was – could have been instrumental in the development of an overly sexualised and entitled approach to women which became problematic as he grew older.

Comments John's experience is a little different to the others, insofar as he reminds us of the cultural, social, and political differences that influence how we interpret behaviour: something that so obviously would have been understood by us as abuse if the perpetrator had been a man was not experienced (or interpreted) as overtly difficult by John, but may nevertheless have caused considerable problems for him in later life.

These brief vignettes of victim to perpetrator narratives provide us with a glimpse of what might be happening. Although incomplete and overly simplified, there are clues here that there may be a specific combination of factors that raise the risk of a victim to perpetrator pathway.

A theoretical model for thinking about the pathway from victim to perpetrator

How might one explain the connection between childhood sexual abuse and committing sexual offences in adulthood? Most of us intuitively understand that victimisation experiences are likely to be psychologically damaging in some way; furthermore, although our condemnation of those who commit sexual offences can cloud our thinking, it is also possible to accept that perpetrators are also, in some way, psychologically disturbed at the time they offend. However, connecting these two 'psychological facts' requires a theoretical understanding to provide an explanatory narrative. There is no one single explanation that suffices, but a number of possible explanations, many of which include ideas about trauma and the way in which trauma interferes with our ability to process and resolve complex emotional and cognitive (thinking) states.

For these reasons, I have chosen to outline simple ideas around the 'compulsion to repeat' and 'identification with the aggressor'. These themes are drawn from psychoanalytic ideas, and help us to understand how it might be possible for an individual to have had a deeply unpleasant or traumatic experience and yet – despite their abhorrence for the behaviour that they experienced as a child – find themselves behaving exactly as their own abuser behaved. As one individual said to me: *'I can't understand it, I ended up doing the same things that were so horrible for me as a kid'*. The ideas are based on the premise that the chronic abuse of a child is a traumatic event which can be overwhelming if there is no strong and containing attachment with a protective and nurturing carer; the child cannot make sense of such abusive experiences – particularly when they are associated with highly conflicting feelings – and is overwhelmed by feelings of anxiety. The 'compulsion to repeat' is linked to the need to take the trauma narrative, but to create a new ending, that is, to master it. In this way, we might understand the victim to perpetrator pathway as repeated unconscious attempts by a sexually traumatised child – as an adult – to reenact and master the original trauma by repeatedly taking the role of perpetrator rather than victim.

If this seems difficult to understand, think of a friend who repeatedly gets into relationships with abusive and belittling men, despite having been deeply disturbed and distressed by her own father's belittling attitude to her when growing up; she repeatedly muses on her apparent inability to refrain from being attracted to 'bad boys', and seems to think that if she can 'just love them enough', they will change. Alternatively, think of those who have experienced a sudden and untimely bereavement; grief reactions in response to a traumatic event are multilayered, but often those who are bereaved in this way find themselves preoccupied with retracing the events leading up to death, pursuing every detail in way that actually helps them unconsciously to process an event that might otherwise be emotionally overwhelming.

'Identification with the aggressor' has the same roots in trauma, as the 'compulsion to repeat', but in this instance, the adult strives to avoid acknowledging the terrible feelings of helplessness or fear experienced as a child, and deals with such feelings by locating them in their victim (when an adult) and attacking them. We see this sometimes in some rape offences when a man savagely attacks a woman and reports being enraged by her fear and excited by his control over her; and we saw it in the vignette of Harry when he unconsciously imposed his anger at his mother onto his partner, and then attacked her (albeit indirectly). We all do this in much more minor ways; for example, most of us can recall a time when we felt bad about ourselves but instead of owning our own feelings, we found ourselves getting angry with someone else – perhaps blaming them – and in doing so, feeling better about ourselves temporarily.

Having introduced ideas of trauma, it may be helpful to pause and consider the nature of trauma, given that it is a widely used word that could perhaps be misleading. Box 5.2 outlines some definitions. Trauma is focused primarily on abnormal events that any 'average person' might find frightening or disturbing; however, in order not to overuse or misuse the word, it is important to consider events that are potentially life-threatening. This is easy to understand when we consider a car crash, major surgery, or a brutal rape by a stranger; it is more complicated to understand when we consider childhood experiences of chronic sexual abuse. However, as was explained in Chapter 2, such experiences do constitute a threat to our survival if we think in evolutionary terms: attachment is crucially important to species where the offspring remain heavily dependent on the nurturing of carers, if they are to survive until independence. A combination of a failure in attachment (what we call insecure attachment) and the complex trauma triggers the same biological responses – fight/flight responses – as a physically life-threatening event.

BOX 5.2

Trauma

Simple trauma is perhaps a misleading term, but refers to the emotional response to a single event – likely to be straightforward to define – that is externally imposed on the individual, and which is experienced as deeply disturbing, shocking, or overwhelming and as a threat to life or bodily/psychological integrity.

Complex trauma incorporates the above ingredients but relates to the psychological and emotional impact on children who have repeatedly experienced neglect or physical or sexual abuse either early in childhood or for a long time in childhood, possibly caused by an important attachment figure.

Frank's story

Frank was a 48-year-old man who had come out of prison a year earlier after serving a seven-year prison sentence for the sexual assault of a 11-year-old boy; I met him after he had moved from a probation hostel to his own flat and was still under the supervision of the probation service, although he was due to conclude his period 'on licence' (probation supervision) in the next couple of months. His progress in the community had been fairly smooth, but the probation officer was concerned that although Frank had a good understanding of his offending behaviour and its impact on his victims, he lacked insight into the more complex emotional and relationship issues that seemed to be underpinning his offending. Frank was also keen to be referred for further psychological help, as he was anxious about the impending conclusion of his time with probation and wanted the security of some additional support longer term. So I met with Frank in my outpatient clinic, and we embarked upon a period of therapeutic work together that lasted for around two years.

Frank had been to court for sexual offences on three separate occasions between the ages of 24 and 42. On the first occasion, as a young adult, he had been convicted of indecent exposure having exposed his penis to a teenage girl in the park as she was walking home from school. For this offence he received a fine, and the matter was closed. Some years later, aged around 31, Frank – having trained as a teacher in information technology and programming – was convicted of an offence of indecent assault on one of his 13-year-old male pupils; he had offered the victim extra support after school to help him catch up with class work, and during this time, had developed their relationship so that he was eventually able to kiss the boy and then fondle his penis. The victim did not disclose the abuse on the first occasion, but told his mother after the second occasion, and Frank was convicted and sentenced to a three-year community order with an expectation that he would participate in a probation-run group intervention for convicted sex offenders. Nowadays, this may appear to be a rather lenient outcome – and indeed, it is most unlikely now that an offender such as Frank, with a prior sexual conviction, would receive a community sentence – but all those years ago, it was a quite common sentencing outcome. Frank participated in the group work programme and was generally cooperative; but with hindsight, he acknowledged that his motivation to desist from offending was half-hearted at the time, and he was emotionally very immature and rather out of his depth in the group. Nevertheless, he completed his community sentence and apparently did not offend for another nine years. His third appearance at court for sexual offending was at the age of 40: Frank had been forbidden from ever teaching again following his previous conviction, and he had picked up self-employed work over the years, sometimes as a gardener or handyman, and at other times as a computer repairer. Nearer to the time that he reoffended, he had developed a heavy drinking habit, and this began to interfere with his ability to obtain and sustain work. With hindsight, it was possible to track the way in which Frank's life had become increasingly isolated, and how his increased intake of alcohol only served to exacerbate his depressed and bitter feelings. The final set of offences occurred when he became friendly with a family who lived down his street; initially he had repaired the household computer, but later he helped out the family with household repairs, and some babysitting of the two boys. The family trusted him, and were particularly grateful for the way in which he bonded with their younger son who had some behavioural difficulties and had been unresponsive to their efforts to manage him. The victim – the younger boy – was aged about 11 when the sexual abuse started, and it continued for several months before the boy felt able to tell a teacher at school, who in turn, contacted the police.

Having received a substantial prison sentence on this last occasion, Frank really started to reflect on his life and the choices he was making about his behaviour. His health deteriorated in prison and for the first time he contemplated the very real and unedifying possibility of dying in prison if he continued to offend. In his view though, the turning point came one day when '*I looked in the mirror and saw a fat and balding bloke, and questioned, am I really sure that I'm sexually attractive to ten year olds?*' He decided to participate in the prison sex offender programme, and this time, put his heart and soul into it, emerging six months later with a markedly changed attitude towards his offending, his responsibility for what occurred, and the impact on his victims. He had taken a constructive attitude toward others in the group, and often helped them with their 'cognitive distortions' – the commonly encountered minimisations and justifications that provided them with excuses to continue offending, and masked their feelings of shame. He was hard on himself as well as others, and continued with this rigorously self-disciplined attitude through into the community.

The Frank who presented himself at my outpatient clinic was, I felt, an individual who had experienced a rather evangelical conversion after the sex offender programme that led to a set of appropriate but rigidly held negative views about himself and his offending. This was helpful to some extent in terms of maintaining his risk to others at a low level in the short term; however, longer term, it was important that he develop an understanding of himself at a more emotional level. This was not something that came easily to him as he was not an expressive individual, but also he rigorously rejected any exploration – or indeed explanation – that appeared to excuse his behaviour. The question is often raised as to whether past trauma and early life events need to be discussed in therapy in order for meaningful behaviour change to be achieved? The answer is sometimes no and sometimes yes – an unhelpful response, but one that reflects the complexity of the decision! Talking in depth about profoundly disturbing trauma experiences can sometimes reduce an individual's ability to cope and increase the risk they might pose to others; many therapies for such individuals focus on interpersonal difficulties and coping skills in the present, rather than exploring the past. However, in Frank's case there were two reasons for exploring his emotional development in more detail: first, his offending was intermittent, by which I mean that there were long periods when he seemed never to think about sex in relation to children; our discussions led me to conclude that he was only strongly driven to offend at times when he felt emotionally fragile – for example, after his mother died, and when he became acutely isolated and depressed – but he lacked insight into the meaning of these triggers. Second, I was aware that Frank had been seriously sexually abused as a child, although interestingly he denied that this experience was abusive, nor that it was relevant to his offending. Without quite knowing where the problem lay or exactly what it signified, I felt intuitively that this trauma narrative contained within it an important key to understanding why he offended.

As already intimated, it took some time for Frank to be able to talk with any meaningful insight into his childhood development and the nature of his complex trauma stemming from childhood. Inevitably our sessions would move from consideration of the past to the here and now – checking for risks, talking about his everyday responses to others in his limited network of relationships – and then to planning for the future: this involved working on what a reasonable quality of life might look like for Frank, one that might enable him to build resilience for those times of difficulty when he might be at risk for offending. Progress, in relation to past events, was clearly facilitated by our developing relationship; that is, Frank learnt gradually that I could be relied upon, not only to turn up regularly, but that I did what I said I would do, and that my observations were designed to be helpful to him rather than to further my own agenda (something of huge relevance, given the narrative set out below). For someone who has been chronically abused as a child, it is not enough to point out the individual's difficulty with trust to effect change, but the therapist has to earn trust in a painstaking fashion. This includes managing times when I, as therapist, was less than perfect; being fallible and being able to talk about it is more important than being near perfect and taking perfection for granted. So we ambled towards insight and understanding, taking many detours and arriving at dead ends before finding a path that seemed to head towards our destination. Frank allowed himself to be pushed outside his comfort zone of rational black and white thinking, and I dropped my language of abuse and trauma, and learned to talk in terms that mirrored Frank's experiences of love and relating.

The story that emerged was one of emotional neglect, abuse, deception, and trauma. Frank was one of two children, although his sister was much older than him; they lived with their mother, their father having left the family home to go working and travelling with the Merchant Navy. For the first five years of his life, he recalled his mother threatening repeatedly *'when your father returns you'll be in trouble'*, but by the time he attended primary school, all talk of his father seemed to fade away, except for the occasional furious comment *'you're just like him'*. Frank's abiding impression of his mother was that she did not like him, and her hostility appeared to be linked to the fact that he took after his father in looks (although perhaps not in personality), and she was very bitter at having been abandoned by him. His sister, by his reckoning, was greatly favoured by his mother, and their bond – an occasional joke as they shared their contempt for the *'uselessness of men'*, and an enviable companionship in completing some of the domestic tasks together – excluded him still further. Frank was a rather timid and studious boy, although not particularly academically able; at school, he seemed to be a target for bullies who considered him to be a *'sissy'* and considered him an *'ass-kisser'* for seeking out the teachers for approval rather than joining in with his peers. He found it difficult to make friends, not being good at sport, and his mother discouraged play dates after school, as being disruptive and unproductive.

For a fairly brief period of time around the age of 9 or 10, Frank's mother attended evening classes in order to improve her chances of promotion at work; given that his sister was now working full-time, a neighbour was drafted into babysit for Frank. This babysitter – a girl in her late teens – was a friend of his sister, and treated him with the same contempt as he felt his sister did. However, the babysitter also sexually abused him on a handful of occasions; for example, instructing him in a fierce tone of voice to play with his penis whilst she inspected his small erection and belittled him for it. Her motives were unclear, although it is possible that she was simply using Frank for sexual experimentation, enjoying the control she had over him at these times. Frank's experience at the time was that these incidents were terrifying and humiliating – painful emotionally and physically – and he recounted the abuse in the therapy room with an expression of anger that was still very live for him.

It was interesting to contrast Frank's account of the babysitter with his demeanour when talking about his '*relationship*' with the scoutmaster. He joined the scouts at the age of 11, and described this in rather idealised terms as '*paradise*' and as '*a haven from my horrible home life*'. As a scout, he found a substitute family where he felt valued and part of a group; he understood the rules and the structure, and found his enthusiasm for '*doing well*' was praised rather than derided. Although Frank did not quite put it in these terms, it was my feeling that the scouts provided an alternative model of masculinity for him that avoided being dismissed as '*sissy*' or overly macho. Frank was sexually abused by the scoutmaster over a period of around two years; his description was that '*I fell in love ... and he loved me in return. ... Yes it was physical, that was what he wanted and I wanted to please him.... [I]t was the way in which we expressed our love for each other*'. A further important component of the sexual abuse was Frank's intense friendship with the scoutmaster's son who was also part of the scout unit, and was sometimes present and also victimised when Frank was being abused. Frank described this relationship as '*he was the brother I had longed to have ... my soul mate. ... [W]e understood each other completely.... [T]here was none of that competitive edge that one has with other boys.... [W]e both loved his dad ... and were loved by him – equally I felt*'. In our therapy sessions, it was months before Frank was able to describe his relationship with the scoutmaster in a more realistic fashion, and he found it extremely painful to do so: '*.I do admit that he used techniques to control me, I can see that now.... I was looking for a father figure and he made sure that he was that person.... [T]here were bribes, being taken on a trip, getting rather generous gifts at Christmas and so on.... [B]ut the real bribes were emotional, 'cos he made me feel like the chosen one, the special one, he picked me out of everyone there*'. The sexual acts themselves seemed to be neither particularly pleasurable to Frank nor particularly distasteful, although he could no longer recall the first few occasions; he was adamant that the abuse '*started after we were already very close and loving, it just seemed the natural next step with him leading the way ... mostly oral sex on each other, mutual masturbation. ... At first I don't think there was any sexual pleasure but as I got a little older, I seem to remember getting erections and a nice warm feeling*'.

When Frank first talked about the scoutmaster, he spoke of the abuse ending '*because he said that other boys needed his love, I had his son's friendship and could find my own source of love with others.... He said it was important that we weren't selfish.... It was painful but he knew best and was probably right*'.

Listening to this account, the reader may feel as cynical as I did at that moment. It seemed to me that Frank was being dropped by his abuser around the onset of puberty when he was becoming less attractive as a target and was easily fobbed off with falsehoods. I recall being fairly angry in the session and expressing my negative feelings towards Frank's abuser; he was resistant to my narrative at the time, but months later was able to reflect on this and say '*I can't say I'm angry with him, not even now ... because if I'm angry then I have to acknowledge that he never loved me, that he simply used me for his own sordid sexual lusts ... and if he never loved me, then I'm left with nothing... I'm just an empty shell*'.

In reality, at the age of 13, Frank had barely any further sexual contact with the scoutmaster, and his feelings about this were put to one side as he remained very close to the scoutmaster's son. However, after the long summer break, expecting to resume his scout activities, Frank was told at school that the unit had broken up and been dissolved, and the scoutmaster and his family had moved away. Disbelieving the situation, he said that he went to their house but found it empty, and he recalled running into the local woods and hiding in the bushes for hours, weeping desperately. Frank found it difficult to know exactly what he was weeping for, as he was not able to disentangle the loss of the scouts as his 'real' family, from the love and caresses of the scoutmaster, or the intense feeling of closeness to his '*soul mate*'.

Frank never told anyone of his experiences of sexual abuse at the hands of the teenage neighbour or the scoutmaster until after he received a long custodial sentence in his 40s. In his teenage years, he was beset with anxieties about his sexual orientation and wanted desperately to be heterosexual; he made tentative and largely unsuccessful efforts to date female peers through until his late 20s. Alcohol was a prop and enabled him to overcome distaste at sexual intimacy with women on a temporary basis, but relationships with women fizzled out largely on account of his failure to communicate at an emotional level. His understanding of his first offence of indecent exposure with a young female victim was that this was a *'cry for help'*, an irrational attempt to *'prove I was normal, my masculinity was not in doubt'*. His sexual offence against a male pupil when he was a teacher in his 30s was triggered by the death of his mother, which raised long buried feelings of anger and bitterness towards her. He later said that he saw in the victim *'a means of seeking solace. ... I felt so...so agitated, I was soothed by his presence, we understood each other and at the time I felt he was able to comfort me ... at least I felt it was him at the time, but now I think it was just the physical touch that comforted me'*. Although he tried hard to refocus his life following the second conviction, Frank never managed to achieve the structure and stability that he needed in order to put his mother's death behind him. Always isolated, he became increasingly aware of an intense state of *'aloneness'* and drank heavily to try and fill the emptiness inside him.

Frank was clearer that the third conviction represented something of a reenactment of his own experiences of abuse with the scoutmaster: *'I saw in the boy a kindred spirit, someone who was misunderstood and had not found his place in life, and I was able to help him, to show him the way. ... Yes it became sexual – lust if I'm honest – but at first it was an intense feeling of closeness and communication, we really understood each other'*. Looking in from the outside, the cynical viewer might insist that Frank groomed the victim of his third conviction from the outset, targeting a family who were vulnerable to his manipulations. However, these words – grooming, targeting, manipulation – can be problematic and lazy descriptors for perpetrator behaviour that has layers of complexity; even though when we think of sexual offending from the victim's experience, the terms are accurate. Frank was all too ready to describe himself as 'grooming the victim' in his enthusiasm to condemn his past behaviour – and there is also a satisfaction for the observer in being able to condemn his motives with such evocative descriptors. However, there are risks in doing so, as we fail to appreciate the underlying emotional drivers for his offending that cannot be undone with glib responses.

Concluding Frank's story

How might we sum up Frank's pathway from victim to abuser? It was certainly not predetermined solely by his biological make-up in terms of personality traits or some sort of inherited 'deviant sexual orientation' – or at least we have little evidence for this driving his behaviour. Nor could we say that it was inevitable that he would become a perpetrator of sexual offences as a result of his early hostile matriarchal family environment, or by his abuse by the neighbour or the abuse by the scoutmaster; yet all these ingredients were a necessary component of the pathway. We need to include his timidity, his social difficulties in adolescence, the lack of a desirable skill or alternative source of self-esteem, his lack of confidence with women, alcohol as a prop for feelings of inadequacy and loneliness; and then we need to consider whether the offences would still have happened if his mother had not died when she did, or if he had had a rich and fulfilling work and leisure life?

At the heart of our understanding of Frank's story lies a trauma; admittedly there are multiple traumas, but there is one, in my view, that dominated his pathway to offending. The primary trauma from which he was never able to recover was the deception perpetrated by the scoutmaster that ended with him being abandoned; that is, the lie that he was loved and cherished by his abuser as a specially chosen individual, rather than the truth – he was one of a series of innocent boys who was used, abused, and dumped. With the physical disappearance of the scoutmaster's family, Frank had to resort to frantic efforts to shield himself from this realisation – he had no loving experiences or secure attachments that could fill the hole left by the acknowledgement of this key deception; he had no intimacy skills with his peers that could provide him with alternative routes to closeness or affection. As a result, his adult life – when stable – was a bleak one characterised by an absence of closeness to others; when unstable, he was drawn back into the original trauma, frantically seeking out boys with whom he could recapture a sense of both lost and idealised intimacy. If we think in terms of the compulsion to repeat, I would suggest that, unconsciously, he tried to master his original trauma by repeating and reversing the outcome; that is, ensuring he would be the one in control, the one who used, abused, and abandoned.

Where is Frank now, 12 years further on and in his 60s? Living independently in the community, and staying in touch occasionally with services – just touching base at times when he feels a little insecure or anxious. He has decided that he is probably homosexual in orientation, and has come to terms with this to the extent that he acknowledges it but prefers to be celibate. He attends Alcoholics Anonymous, although he has not drunk now for almost 20 years; he finds the 12 steps helpful and the warm acceptance of the group meetings very compelling (although no one knows the nature of his conviction). He remains committed to helping others who have sexual convictions, and has found constructive meaning and value in volunteering with ex-offenders, the only setting where his conviction is known and accepted. As far as we can tell in a society that is highly risk-vigilant and closely monitored, he has not reoffended. His life does not have the richness that comes with diverse and close relationships, but it has structure and purpose; Frank's view is *'if they put me in my coffin knowing that I have hurt no more people, then that is success enough for me'*. He may be right, but in my view, Frank underplays what he has achieved in recent years: facing up to the past, as victim and perpetrator, takes courage and strength; and his efforts to manage himself and to give back to the community come from a desire to acknowledge the harm he has caused. He may never have had the experience of love, but he has come to know what it is to be part of something and to be valued.

Further reading

The Independent Inquiry into Child Sexual Abuse is ongoing in the United Kingdom. Unusually, the Inquiry has invested heavily in research, and their website provides reliable and informative reports on issues of close interest to the Inquiry. Information can be found here: https://www.iicsa.org.uk/publications

For academic publications looking at the pathway from victim to perpetrator, the following two articles are relevant:

Craissati, J., McClurg, G., & Browne, K. (2002). Characteristics of perpetrators of child sexual abuse who have been sexually victimised as children. *Sexual Abuse: A Journal of Research and Treatment, 14(3)*, 225–240

Craissati, J., & Beech, A. (2004). The characteristics of a geographical sample of convicted rapists: sexual victimisation and compliance in comparison to child molesters. *Journal of Interpersonal Violence, 19 (3)*, 225–240.

Perhaps of tangential relevance as it does not touch on forensic cases, the following book is a highly regarded volume that articulates complex psychoanalytic ideas for the non-analyst in accessible and highly readable ways.

Malan, D. H. (1995). Individual Psychotherapy and the Science of Psychodynamics. Oxford: Butterworth-Heinemann.

There are numerous books on men who commit sexual offences. A good starting point would be the following edited volume:

Beech, A., Craig, L.A., & Browne, K.D. (2009). Assessment and Treatment of Sex Offenders: A Handbook. West Sussex: John Wiley & Sons Ltd.

Kevin, Len, and Mark's story 6

Getting to grips with risk assessment

This chapter focuses exclusively on the task of risk assessment: the prediction of future sexual or physical violence in those individuals who have already been convicted of at least one act of violence. Previous chapters have largely focused on the question of 'why' – understanding why individuals commit serious crimes of violence from a psychological point of view; in this chapter, we consider 'whether' such an offence will happen again. The task is relatively straightforward, the goal being *to achieve as great a degree of accuracy in predicting violent outcomes as possible*. Accuracy, in this instance, means that we need to identify as many likely reoffenders as possible within our risk assessment (true positives, see Box 6.1) without scooping up too many non-reoffenders into the same high-risk net (false positives). Emotionally, we are biased towards trying to avoid missing any reoffenders (false negatives), but in terms of human rights and social justice, it is important not to deny low-risk individuals (true negatives) the opportunity to lead offence-free lives in the community.

Before going any further, it may be helpful to be clear about our risk terminology:

- **Risk assessment**, as described above, is the process of collating the relevant risk information to help determine the likelihood of a specific outcome.
- **Risk judgements** refer to the analysis arising from the assessment, that may or may not require evidence-based adjustments in response to specific circumstances.

BOX 6.1

Accuracy in risk assessment

True positives: correctly identified individuals who go on to reoffend
False positives: incorrectly identified individuals who are predicted to reoffend but do not
True negatives: correctly identified individuals who will not go on to reoffend
False negatives: incorrectly identified individuals who are predicted not to reoffend but in fact do reoffend

- **Risk management** is the planned response to the risk judgement, which usually involves strategies for minimising risk concerns and promoting strengths/protective features.

Arguably, we are living in an era where a large proportion of the public – and politicians – have become disillusioned with expertise; certainly, with social media, it seems that not only does everyone feel able to express an opinion but that everyone's opinion is of equal value and weight in matters that may sit outside their expertise. The experts have to take a good deal of responsibility for this state of affairs, having failed to communicate with the public in ways that engage and have meaning. Therefore, the aim of this chapter is to redress that situation by communicating the science of risk assessment in a way that enables interested others to understand – and more importantly, to have confidence in – our approach to risk judgements. In emphasising the word 'science' when referring to good risk assessments, I want to acknowledge the limitations of our state of knowledge currently and the inherent difficulties in predicting human behaviour; nevertheless, there is a science to the process, and a track record of empirical study within the social sciences. Here, by science, we mean that our judgements must be based on the known, consistent, and published evidence base, although – as will be demonstrated later in the chapter – it is difficult to avoid the pull of emotions in this task. For example, at the time of writing this chapter, a terrorist incident in south London follows on from a dreadful terrorist attack at London Bridge two months earlier; both perpetrators were automatically released from prison sentences for prior related offences. The public may well consider, as a result, that convicted terrorists pose a high risk of reoffending, not least because the public will have no idea of how many convicted terrorists have been released and gone on to lead pro-social lives. Expert testimony – for example, that around 10% or less of such offenders perpetrate further similar offences when back in the community – does nothing to assuage public concern at such times. Indeed, such statistics seem offensive when we are still reeling from the enormity of the crime, and the devastation that it has wrecked on victims and their families. The dramatic loss of public confidence that is associated with a serious further offence – committed whilst under the supervision of the authorities – is palpable, and shared by those likely devastated practitioners who have been responsible for the management of such offenders.

However, we make judgements about risk all the time in our daily lives; when we get in a car, smoke cigarettes, drink to excess, go scuba diving, take a trip in a helicopter, cross the road. We understand that there is a risk of harm (even death) in all these activities, but we make judgements about relative likelihood of harm or benefit to us, and tolerate the risk. This becomes a much more difficult societal conversation when thinking about the tolerance of risk for violent crime: if we accept that there is no possibility of zero risk in this field, then there has to be a discussion about what degree of risk is tolerable. For some risks, we engage in errors of thinking – distorted reasoning – that enables us to tolerate a risk by miscalculating it. For example, many years ago when conducting some research with women who were in relationships with convicted sex offenders, I was struck by their calculation of the risk to their children. When asked 'how likely are sex offenders to reoffend?', they mostly judged the risk to be around 70–90% likelihood; when then asked immediately afterwards 'how likely is it that your partner will reoffend?', they estimated the risk to be 0–10%. The women could not be dismissed as 'bad mothers' or as 'stupid'; they were simply trying to manage the cognitive and emotional task of resolving the tension between an uncomfortable risk and a longed for benefit to the family.

Risk tolerance is a social and political decision; the role of the expert is simply to offer the clearest and most accurate possible risk assessment with associated advice. For example, if we consider how the Parole Board operates in England and Wales; it is often the case that a number of practitioners – usually a probation officer and sometimes a psychologist – provide a risk assessment, whilst an independent panel of Parole Board members – with public protection foremost in their mind – make the decision regarding release. We have fairly accurate and consistent figures for the outcome of Parole Board release decisions for the first three years following release: for example, the Annual Report of the Parole Board (2017/18) reports 4,291 individuals were recommended for release from prison that year and, separately, 31 cases were considered by the committee that reviews grave reoffending. Figures for other years are remarkably similar, and suggest overall that less than 1% of all serious offenders released by the Parole Board commit further sexual or violent offences during the first three years of leaving prison. If we consider that the Parole Board only deals with those prisoners who have long determinate prison sentences and all those with indeterminate (life) sentences – both of which are more likely to be associated with the most series crimes and the most challenging of offenders – this is an outstandingly good record for a public institution. Yet can we say that our risk tolerance for violent reoffending is 1% when each one of those 30 or so reoffences is a devastating event for those concerned?

Understanding the context for considering risk

Our approach to risk assessment tends to focus on the traits of the offender – behaviours, thoughts, and feelings associated with increased likelihood of a repetition – but we may make mistakes if we fail to take into account the context in which offending occurs. This is easier to understand if we consider an example that is less emotive than those associated with violent crimes. Consider a mother of two young children who has a car crash as she drives the children to the child minder: she is tired after yet another disturbed night's sleep, and although the route is familiar to her, she is distracted by the squabbling children in the back of the car as she approaches a junction in the road. She drives across the junction – the markings somewhat faded over time – without checking carefully enough for other cars, and drives into the side of a car that is approaching from the right just at that moment. The other driver has right of way and is driving within the speed limit, therefore the mother is responsible for the accident in which both drivers are shaken up but not seriously hurt. Our risk assessment is focused on the future likelihood of the mother having a further accident – that is, will it happen again – and we may well decide that her lack of sleep and distractibility were key risk factors in determining the accident. This seems to be relatively straightforward, until we consider that the woman has driven this route around 200 times previously and, on a significant number of occasions has been both tired and distracted without incurring an accident. How powerful are these risk factors, therefore, in determining future risk even though they were clearly implicated in the original crash? Might it be that the victim's behaviour (the driver who was hit) – being in the wrong place at the wrong time – contributed to the crash even though we are clear that this driver was not in any way responsible for the incident? Or could it be that the unclear road markings made a significant contribution to the incident, again without reducing the woman's responsibility for the crash? In order to calculate the risk of reoccurrence more accurately, we need to consider the evidence base for risk associated with driving, and this is the approach taken by actuaries who work in the car insurance industry. Actuaries use mathematics and statistics to study uncertain future events, and help in developing formulae for calculating insurance premiums. A very simplified interpretation of actuarially determined risks in car accidents suggests that young people – particularly young men – and single people pose a higher risk; women who are married and over the age of 25 are a particularly low-risk group of individuals. Applying this statistical knowledge to our example of the mother with two young children – and taking into account the fact that she is probably driving a reliable family car – we should probably assume that she falls into a low-risk category, and that the identified risk factors – sleeplessness and distractibility – are indeed factors with only a modest link to the likelihood of a further road traffic accident. Furthermore, if we take into account the shock of the accident on the woman driver, and the likelihood of her being extremely cautious in future, then we may conclude that the risk of another accident is negligible. Clearly, if this particular road junction has been the site of previous accidents with other drivers, our risk management approach might be to recommend an improvement by the Local Authority to the road markings at the junction, but an intervention with the driver herself does not seem to be warranted.

However, before we can leave this example, we need to consider whether we would arrive at the same conclusion if we knew that the woman had had a car accident on two previous occasions, in different locations, as this would seem to suggest a pattern of behaviour that might indicate an underlying problem that was increasing the risk. Consider, for example, a situation in which the mother was found to have a problem with heavy alcohol use, and that she was hungover on the morning of the accident, or that she had previously been noted to drive erratically and make impulsive and poor decisions in relation to her judgement when driving. These are all traits or behaviours that might lead us to consider her as higher risk of a further accident, despite her demographics placing her in a low-risk category. Here, our adjustment of the risk is also evidence based because we are familiar with the significant role of alcohol that is implicated in road traffic accidents. We also have one further consideration to make: is the likelihood of a future car accident closely linked to the seriousness of harm that results from the accident? In other words, whether distractibility and tiredness – or indeed, heavy alcohol use the night before – predict a fatal car accident. Probably the single most important predictor of serious harm is whether or not everyone involved was wearing their seat belt, although it is likely that the safety record of the cars involved, the angle of impact, and the speed of the cars at the time of impact are all salient factors.

This example, in general terms, leads us to some important conclusions:

- There is a difference between identifying contributory factors to the original incident and concluding that these factors will determine future risk.
- Clarity regarding responsibility for an incident should be considered independently of the risk assessment.
- For those individuals who fall into a low-risk category on the basis of the known evidence, there is little indication for a personalised intervention (although it may be beneficial to consider the environment in which the incident was able to occur).
- The factors that are involved in an assessment of likelihood of reoccurrence are probably very different to the factors that are associated with the seriousness of harm.

The risk assessment of men with histories of convictions for serious violence

Our consideration of the above scenario sets the scene for the main focus of this chapter: taking an objective and evidence-based approach to predicting future violence in men who have already been convicted of violent crimes. To this end, three case vignettes are set out below; to make the task manageable, all three men have been convicted of physically violent (rather than sexually violent) offences, and the information provided is succinct but sufficient to enable a reasonable risk assessment to be undertaken. Kevin is an individual who has committed offences of domestic violence against his wife; Len has been convicted of the murder of a woman who was a stranger to him, and Mark assaulted a shopkeeper in the course of an armed robbery.

Step one is to read the three vignettes, and to consider what level of future risk the individual might pose when released into the community. Focus on the likelihood of violence, rather than non-violent general offending, and consider risk over a time period of around four years in the community. This timescale is often chosen as we know that most reoffending – if it is to occur – is likely to happen within a few years of release. Make a note to yourself of all the features of the vignette that are influencing your risk assessment; however, if you find the task overly complicated, try and focus on the two or three features that you feel are most salient to the risk assessment.

Case vignettes

Kevin (aged 37) has served six years of an eight-year custodial sentence for three convictions for assault (actual bodily harm – ABH) and one of grievous bodily harm (GBH) with intent to harm (GBH Section 18) on his wife of five years. There was a further allegation of rape made against him by his wife, to which he pleaded not guilty, and this was dropped before coming to court. The offences took place over a six-month period as the relationship – which had previously been fairly stable – was deteriorating. His wife was making plans to leave him, due to his unreasonably controlling and threatening behaviour. Neighbours had also reported that he was argumentative with them at times and had a threatening demeanour.

Kevin had been a prolific offender between the ages of 16 and 26, often committing burglaries with his peers, as well as some drugs offences and driving offences. He had also been a heavy drinker and drug user, although these problems had greatly improved in the couple of years prior to his current offence.

As a child, he witnessed his father's repeated violence towards his mother, and often tried to intervene to protect his mother, although he ended up being hit as a result. His father left when he was aged 7 years. At the age of 11, Kevin was taken into care, and later learned that this had been because his mother worked as a prostitute, and he was often neglected by her. He remained in care until an adult, and developed a marked anti-authoritarian stance, continuously rebelling.

After a calm period of about four years in the community prior to this sentence, Kevin is now struggling in prison: during this sentence he has received 15 adjudications (prison hearings), mostly for disobeying orders, although he has been verbally threatening to other prisoners on two occasions and he threatened to head-butt an officer who he felt was '*taking the piss*'. He has a prickly relationship with his female probation officer. He has completed the Healthy Relationships Programme in prison, with mixed reports. He admits to struggling with feelings of dependency and a fear of abandonment in intimate relationships, but he is resistant to exploring alternative means of managing his feelings in any detail.

Len (aged 51) received a life sentence of 25 years previously for the murder of a 31-year-old woman. On the day of the offence, he had been drinking heavily instead of going into work. He was feeling angry after a row with his father the night before. He was walking home around 6 p.m. when he noticed that he was going in the same direction as the woman in front. Without any conscious planning, he grabbed the woman from behind, dragged her into the bushes, and strangled her. He recalled watching her face contort until she lost consciousness. He was unsure whether she was truly dead, so picked up a heavy stone which was lying nearby and smashed it down upon her head. Realising what he had done, he went home, and the next day gave himself up to the police.

At trial, it was mentioned that Len had once lost his temper with a new boss at work and been very verbally threatening, but this had not led to any physical violence. He has no previous convictions.

Len described himself as the black sheep of the family: his mother had always wanted a girl, and used to buy him dolls for toys and allow his hair to grow long. When 6 years old, longed-for twin sisters were born, he felt that his mother subsequently ignored him. His father was a strict and critical man who made it clear that Terry had failed him, but was never physically violent. School was uneventful and Terry was described as quiet and obedient, and moderately bright. Since leaving school, he worked as a sales assistant and then manager for eight years until his index offence. He had had no sexual relationships.

In prison, Len's behaviour has been very good, and he held a job as a cleaner for much of the time as well as obtaining further academic and vocational qualifications. He was able to speak in great detail about his early life and the offence, although played down his negative feelings towards his family; he said he felt very low when thinking about the victim and the offence. He was described as a stickler for accuracy and tended to make multiple formal complaints in relation to prison procedures. Male professionals considered him to have changed considerably since the offence, his female field probation officer experienced him as overly controlling.

Mark (aged 26) was convicted of armed robbery and assault, and had received a six-year custodial sentence of which he had served four years. On the day of the offence, he had run out of amphetamines and decided to rob a jeweller shop, with the help of a friend as lookout. He took an imitation firearm with him and demanded gold chains and cash off the jeweller, threatening to kill him if he did not comply. The man pressed the shop alarm and Mark panicked, punching him hard in the face and running off.

Mark was first convicted when he was aged 12, and he had accumulated a long string of convictions for taking and driving away, theft, and shoplifting and burglaries. Aged 18, he had served an 18-month sentence for assault on an old school friend he met whilst out drinking in a pub: this occurred whilst he was on probation for an offence of burglary. He offered her a lift home, but outside her flat made a pass at her, which she rebuffed; he became angry and punched her, saying she was a *"teasing c**t"*.

Mark was the youngest of four children. His parents had a turbulent relationship, predominantly because his father was a heavy drinker and often in prison. At school, he found it difficult to concentrate and was disruptive, being suspended once when he was 9 because he hit a teacher. By secondary school he was frequently truanting and fighting with classmates. He did not obtain any qualifications, although he was considered to be bright. He had only ever worked sporadically in casual labouring jobs, not least because he had spent so much time in prison. He had started experimenting with cannabis and glue sniffing in early adolescence, but had developed a dependency on amphetamines and cocaine, which accounted for his thieving. He had had a number of sexual relationships with women, none of which had lasted longer than six months.

In prison, Mark appeared to settle down and his behaviour was reasonable. He participated in a number of relevant group interventions. He was determined that he would avoid old acquaintances who were a bad influence on him, and that he would be careful in future to use drink – and occasionally drugs – on a social basis only. His female probation officer found him to be likeable and was optimistic about his future; his male probation officer found him defensive and hostile and they quickly established an antagonistic relationship.

Step two is to reconsider your risk assessment when informed that that there is one low-risk, one medium-risk, and one high-risk individual within the three vignettes. Consider whether this new information changes your assessment – whether you are able to identify which of the three is low-, medium-, or high-risk – and try to be more specific about which particular factors you believe to be particularly important in influencing your decision. Low-, medium-, and high-risk categories are relative rather than absolute terms: you may not know exactly what percentage of offenders within each category go on to commit further violent offences, but you can rate the vignettes against each other. That is, which of the three offenders are less or more likely than the other two to commit further offences.

Step three is to analyse the risk in relation to the known evidence base, and to test this analysis against your intuitive and/or common sense reasoning. In considering Kevin, Len, and Mark in turn, I will highlight for the reader the common errors in reasoning to which not only the public but also practitioners in the field are prone, as well as laying out in broad terms the reliable risk predictors in each case.

First, I should acknowledge my own assumptions as to the readers' conclusions regarding the vignettes. I think it is likely that more readers struggled to find a low-risk vignette than to find a high-risk vignette, and that thoughts such as 'yes, but what about…' crept into the revision of risk at step two. I also suspect – on the basis of experience – that readers identified far more 'worrying' risk factors than 'reassuring' (often called protective) risk factors; and that readers were reluctant to give up risk factors when asked to be more stringent. We are all naturally inclined to be cautious, risk averse, and anxious not to miss possible risk identifiers. Finally, I assume that readers had different emotional reactions to the three vignettes, and that these emotional responses strongly influenced the approach to the task.

Box 6.2 outlines the key risk factors that are known to have a strong evidence base in considering the future risk of violence. This evidence is dominated by research from North America and Western Europe; there is some limited work to evaluate the relevance and accuracy of standard risk approaches in wider cultural contexts, but it is important to exercise caution in making assumptions about diverse cultures and risk. Practitioners in the field of mental health and criminal justice no longer rely simply on experience and

BOX 6.2

Known and reliable risk factors in assessing future violence

1. **Age**
   Most offenders desist from violence with age, with the likelihood reduced very considerably from the age of 30 onward, continuing to decrease still further over time. Age is considered to be a static factor, as there is nothing we can do to influence it except for time passing.
2. **Previous convictions**
   Prior offending behaviour is a strong predictor of future violence, although not in itself sufficient to be accurate, particularly as the offender matures. The offender can do nothing to alter these risk factors. An assessment might take into account
   - The number of prior appearances at court for sentencing in relation to violent offences
   - The range of types of prior convictions of any sort
   - The number of general or the number of violent convictions
   - The age at which the first conviction occurred (particularly under the age of 13)
3. **Antisocial traits**
   These include persistent behaviours in various aspects of everyday life that may have started in childhood but have persisted into adulthood:
   - Persistent rule breaking and other irresponsible behaviour
   - Heavy substance misuse generally, or specifically heavy alcohol use
   - A poor track record of maintaining employment and/or relationships
   - Poor compliance with those in authority

4. **Emotional and behavioural controls**
   This area considers anger in particular, but wider emotional states and behaviours are relevant, including
   - Intense unstable emotions
   - The frequency and degree of anger outbursts
   - Impulsive behaviours and poor decision-making in response to strong emotional states
5. **Criminal lifestyle factors**
   This area focuses on associates and choices about lifestyle that support or condone aggressive solutions, and include
   - The nature and range of criminal associates (friends, family members, or peers engaged in criminal activity)
   - The environment that may adversely influence the individual's decisions and behaviours (which might, for example, include the living environment, local gang activity, the choice of drinking venue)

judgement as there is a long tradition of research into such risk judgements and they are invariably shown to be little better than chance in terms of predictive accuracy. Practitioners therefore use scales and structured guidance that is based on a combination of statistical evidence and theoretical ideas rooted in research and evaluation. Such approaches do contain differences – for example, one method might emphasise the number or range of prior convictions, another might emphasise only prior violent convictions – but overall there is considerable overlap between approaches, and these most reliable factors are presented in Box 6.1. As the reader can discern from the table, some of the risk factors are static – that is, they are historical and cannot be changed – whilst others are referred to as dynamic as they can change in response to maturation in the individual, and may be a target for intervention.

The list in Box 6.2 is perhaps as interesting for what it does not include as for what it does include. The reader will note that there is no reference to denial of the offence, or associated themes such as taking full responsibility for what occurred or attitudes towards the offence. Chapter 3 provides a detailed explanation as to why this might be the case, explaining how shame often drives these offence minimisations or rationalisations and is unrelated to risk. Furthermore, the degree of harm is not specified as a risk factor, or the use of weapons, and yet we are rightly concerned regarding the use of weapons. As we saw with the example of the car accident earlier in this chapter, seriousness of harm is often related to factors other than those which are driving the likelihood of a further offence occurring; weapons are undoubtedly linked to the seriousness of harm caused (the outcome), but the evidence suggests that they do not in themselves indicate that violence is more likely to occur.

Kevin is the medium-risk case vignette. At first glance, this seems to negate the undoubted seriousness of his violent behaviour towards his wife. It also seems to contradict the public's understanding of domestic violence as a crime that persists over time, despite court involvement, and that it is inevitably repeated in all intimate relationships. It is also true that Kevin has a significant history of general (non-violent) offending in his late adolescence and early 20s and that he has had significant problems with substance misuse. He could be described as anti-authoritarian and non-compliant, with ongoing temper control problems. We might assume from his disturbed childhood that further domestic violence is inevitable.

However, we need to root our risk assessment, in the first instance, in a general consideration of future risk in convicted domestic violence offenders. Although studies vary, on average around 40% of such individuals are rearrested for further domestic violence offences. It seems difficult to accept this statistic, given the understandable concern regarding the repetitive behaviour of domestic violence offenders, but an idea or assertion that is familiar does not necessarily mean that it is entirely accurate. Despite the accepted caveat that not all offending behaviour is identified by the authorities or disclosed by victims, there are some mitigating factors in Kevin's presentation.

- Kevin is now aged 37, and this is associated with reduction in risk, although caution needs to be applied, as he was violent towards his wife quite late in adulthood (aged 30 or so).
- There is evidence that the violence within the relationship only took place towards the end of a four- to five-year period when the relationship was breaking down; there is no known evidence of prior violence in relationships, and so a repetition cannot be assumed.
- Kevin's strong antisocial background fell into a common pattern in which he began to mature in his late 20s, settling down around the time that he met and then lived with his wife. Growing out of offending is the norm rather than the exception.
- Substance misuse is relevant to risk, but intoxication was not associated with the violence towards his wife, as he had ceased drinking before the violence commenced.
- There is no doubt that controlling and authoritarian behaviour has been a persistent problem within his marital relationship and with others in authority, however – excluding the violent convictions against his wife – he appears to be defiant and on occasion verbally abusive, but

not physically violent. In other words, he can exercise a degree of self-control despite an intimidating demeanour, and has generally done so throughout his life.

- Although it is very uncertain as to whether Kevin has benefited from a relevant intervention in prison and he does seem to lack some emotional insight, these are factors that have an uncertain relationship to future risk.

An assessment of medium risk of future violence does not preclude the need to be extremely cautious about the risk assessment, and to be alert to potentially triggering or risky situations that might arise in future. Sensible risk management approaches, and the outcome for Kevin after a period of time in the community, is discussed below in the final section to this chapter.

Len is the low-risk case vignette. For many, this will seem to be an assertion lacking credibility. How can someone who committed such a shockingly violent and catastrophic offence be considered low risk in future? For many readers, it is the emotive element of the offence that drives their assessment of him being a risk to women in the future. The vignette – as well as that of Mark – is an amended version of vignettes used in a research project to evaluate the role of emotion in estimating risk amongst mental health practitioners; the research showed how even with risk-knowledgeable practitioners, emotions associated with the depiction of violent crimes were much more powerful in influencing risk decisions than known evidence-based factors.[1] It is almost as though by asserting that Len poses a low risk, we are saying that his offence can be forgiven or excused, and we strenuously resist this implication. However, we need to start with some statistics – how many of those convicted of killing someone go on to commit another violent offence of any sort when back in the community? The estimated answer – based on Parole Board figures and also some limited research that follow up such offenders over longer periods of time – suggests that somewhere around 1% commit grave reoffences (of a violent nature). Of course, this is quite different to asserting that those who kill pose such a low risk at the time of their conviction; it is only when released many years later that we are considering the risk assessment. Therefore, with Len, a truly objective and calm consideration of known risk factors suggests the following:

- Len is of a mature age, associated with a very small risk of further violent offending.
- He has no prior convictions of any type.

- There is one known prior occasion in which he lost his temper, but there is no pattern of poor anger control, either in childhood or adulthood. In fact, his history suggests someone of exemplary self-control in general, except for the night before and during the offence.
- He was clearly intoxicated on the day of the offence, but there is no pattern of significant substance misuse.
- There is some indication of hostility towards women, but this is largely implied, as there is no evidence of overt hostile behaviours towards women more generally, including female criminal justice staff.
- Although pedantic and prickly in his demeanour, this seems to be associated with an insistence on others adhering to the rules (and making complaints if this is not done) rather than any rule breaking himself.

In other words, the risk assessment is low on the basis of the absence of any significantly aggravating risk factors. This suggests that Len is someone whose strong self-control and lack of self-awareness led to a rather solitary life associated with limited emotional expression; it was only when brooding resentments in relation to tense family relationships led to a rare moment of alcohol intoxication that he committed a devastating but opportunistic violent offence. Despite – I anticipate – the readers' doubts in this case, such individuals rarely reoffend.

Mark is the high-risk case vignette, and probably the result that least surprised the reader. His profile is unremarkable for its familiarity to those who work in the criminal justice system. He is high risk because he is still relatively young, with a substantial history of offending that commenced at an unusually young age; furthermore, his offending profile is diverse, with a prior violent offence that had a sexual element to it, as well as burglaries and other less serious offences of theft. His behaviour had been problematic from primary school onwards, characterised by impulsivity and an impetuous problem-solving style; his later lifestyle was broadly feckless and erratic, strongly influenced by significant ongoing substance misuse. There is a suggestion – not very clearly stated – that his friends and associates were probably similar to him in behaviour, and he appears to have been breaking rules even when under probation supervision in the past. It is true that in prison Mark's behaviour was greatly improved, despite obvious temptations to engage in antisocial and subversive behaviours with his peers, and the clarity around rules and regulations may well have helped him to focus. A likeable personality is often thought of as a positive trait in an individual, as it facilitates good engagement with others who are motivated to support such individuals; furthermore, his good intentions to manage his use of substances and avoid negative influences were probably sincere within the prison environment but probably not sufficiently thought through to persist out into the community.

Normally, with individuals such as Mark, the likelihood of violent reconviction might be more than 50% in their early to mid-20s, but almost all such individuals do desist from offending over the passage of time; however, Mark's unusually early behavioural problems and early first conviction raise questions as to whether this natural course of desistance is likely to take more time with Mark than with others who have a significantly anti-social profile.

Risk management outcomes for Kevin, Len, and Mark

This chapter has been focused on the task of accurate risk assessment, the reason being that with limited resources, criminal justice agencies always need to prioritise public protection measures according to greatest need, with an emphasis on targeting those features of an individual's risk that are most likely to lead to negative outcomes. There is a level of sophistication to good risk management – a mixture of common sense, evidence-based approaches, and creativity – that cannot be fully explored here, and there are many books on the subject for the interested reader. However, having confidently asserted that Kevin, Len, and Mark are medium-, low-, and high-risk respectively, it is important that we follow them up for a few years to see what happened when they were released into the community.

For Kevin, there were understandable concerns regarding his future involvement in any new intimate relationship, and a close eye was kept on the level of his alcohol intake and any drug use. His probation supervision included the licence condition that he participated in a domestic violence intervention, something that he deeply resented having already completed a similar programme in prison. He was allocated a mature and experienced female probation officer, and it was to her credit that the outcome for Kevin was – ultimately – a positive one. However, his progress was stormy as he reverted to hostile behaviours in response to licence restrictions that he perceived as unfair. He behaved at times in ways that were intended to control and intimidate his probation officer, but she was able to understand the ways in which this presentation was linked to early childhood experiences, and she managed to maintain an honest, firm, but fair approach to his supervision. Unfortunately, after several months, events overtook any progress in the supervisory relationship, because Kevin was discovered to have hidden a new and now reasonably established intimate relationship from his probation officer. He was recalled to prison, in breach of his licence;

furious, he demanded a change in probation officer, but this – sensibly – was refused and he was forced to work through the impasse in their relationship. She recommended his release, and included his new partner in elements of the probation supervision, ensuring that the partner was able to understand the nature of any risks that Kevin might pose to her, and engaging her constructively from time to time when monitoring the risk. Kevin has now been out of prison for around four years, and remains in the same intimate relationship which is sometimes a little stormy but not physically violent; his drinking remains under control, and he has maintained employment for the past two years.

Len has now been out of prison for 12 years, and although his behaviour has been exemplary in terms of compliance with his life licence, the success of his risk management plan has been reliant on strong collaborative working between the forensic mental health service and the probation service. It became clear early on that there were odd aspects to Len's personality – traits of a rather autistic nature (although he did not meet the threshold for autistic spectrum disorder) – which, when coupled with the horrific and unexpected nature of his original offence, worried probation staff who were tasked with managing the risk. Essentially, the forensic mental health team were able to share the burden of responsibility with the probation service, and brought a clinical perspective to the shared task of disentangling Len's risk from his unusual personality traits. Len has responded best to regular but moderately infrequent contact with services, with a good structure to his week of activity that he finds rewarding; on the rare occasions that the predictable structure has broken down, or contact has been too intrusive – for example, with a new probation officer asking probing questions about his fantasy life – Len can become a little irritable. On one occasion, he appeared to slip into depression after a failed attempt at dating – but a quick and supportive response from the rather anxious multi-agency team, together with some antidepressant medication in the short term, quickly led to him settling down. It seems unlikely that Len will ever be able to be fully discharged from services, despite the low nature of the risk; but currently his probation support is less intensive, and he has a more informal and irregular level of contact with mental health services, with a greater level of contact with other ex-offenders who attend informal support groups.

Mark, as predicted, fared worse than Kevin and Len, although the first few months after he was released went quite well. He was referred to the drug and alcohol team for an assessment, and his sentence plan focused on achieving stability in terms of work and housing. His sister's husband had offered work as a garage mechanic at his place of work, and Mark was moving to his mother's house from the Approved Premises. He attended all probation appointments – sometimes he was late, but he always had a reason for this – and spoke with his probation officer of his positive intentions, including helping his mother to decorate her front room and improving his relationship with his sister who had previously refused to have anything to do with him. However, by the end of his first year in the community, Mark's progress seemed to falter: the drug and alcohol team discharged him on the basis that he said that his drug use was non-existent, and all drug screens were negative; somehow, for reasons that were obscure, the job offer evaporated; and it became clear that Mark was only staying occasionally at his mother's house, as he seemed to be sleeping on a series of friends' sofas. His probation officer tightened up supervision expectations, and tried to address these concerns with Mark, but he remained upbeat and reassuring, albeit slightly evasive in response to questions as to how he was spending his time. The probation officer shared her concerns with police in the risk management team, and with her supervisor, but there was no wider intelligence to suggest anything substantial of concern.

However, 15 months after his release, Mark was arrested for attempted murder, along with an associate. The details of this serious further offence seem to be that Mark became embroiled in drug dealing a few months after release, encouraged by his cousin and friends with whom he was staying at times. He began to carry a knife on a fairly habitual basis, because he perceived that he had a need to defend himself, *'not because I was stupid enough to want to use it'*. He had begun to fall into debt on account of taking some of the drugs that he was selling for personal use; on the night of the offence, he and his cousin had just bought some drugs off the victim – another dealer – and decided to return to the victim's house in order to steal the cash that they knew he had on him. An altercation arose, and in the course of the argument, Mark stabbed the victim once in the stomach, and then ran off. At court, Mark received an indeterminate sentence with a tariff (punishment period) of 12 years.

Even with the benefit of hindsight, it is difficult to see what the probation service or the police might have done differently. Unsubstantiated concerns regarding a theoretically high-risk but otherwise unremarkable offender is unlikely to attract a highly expensive surveillance operation; it is possible that more frequent but random drug testing might have identified a growing problem with crack cocaine use, but this is difficult to sustain 15 months after release at a point when probation supervision was due to cease. What Mark's story does highlight is the importance of paying as much if not more attention to the criminal environment – lifestyle and associates – of the individual on probation supervision rather than the personal risk characteristics;

this includes using supervision to attend to the financial benefits of a criminal lifestyle relative to poorly paid legitimate employment.

Summary

The aim of this chapter was not to teach the reader how to conduct a risk assessment, but to explain the process that practitioners follow in order to strive for predictive accuracy, and in doing so, to build public confidence in the process. Of course, not all cases turn out exactly as predicted: although I am confident that Len is low risk, it was always possible that Kevin would punch someone and acquire a new violent conviction; in Mark's case, he will desist from violence one day, there is little doubt, but on this occasion he was simply not ready to make sufficiently radical changes to his image and his lifestyle. To some extent, these three stories also highlight the importance of collaboration in risk management – collaboration between agencies in the case of Len, and collaboration between offender and supervisor in the case of Kevin and Mark. To explain this a little more clearly, Mark's supervisor was reliant to some extent on Mark's willingness to engage honestly with the probation service; his decision to hide all his problematic behaviours and present a false picture of himself meant that the probation officer was unable to support him effectively. In some cases, police intelligence can take the place of a collaborative approach, but in most cases there is simply no intelligence to share. With Kevin, although he hid his intimate relationship from his probation officer and was found out, for the most part he was honestly belligerent and oppositional in supervision! In the struggle of their relationship, they found a way of working together that was ultimately productive.

Finally, we can conclude that emotions inevitably creep into the risk assessment process when we are thinking about violent behaviour, which is why common sense can only take us so far before leading us astray. In each of the three vignettes, the practitioners meeting the individuals had emotional reactions to them; these reactions are important as they add to the evidence source. However, it is important not take these emotional responses too literally as an accurate barometer of risk: is our feeling of hostility towards an individual an indication of violence risk, or is it an expression of our horror at having read about their offence before going into the room; if we experience someone as controlling, is this evidence of him posing a risk to people in authority, or is it the way in which he manages feelings of anxiety at being judged. These enquiries will be relevant to understanding an individual, but may or may not be linked to their risk assessment.

Note

1. Blumenthal, S., Huckle, C., Czornyj., Craissati, J., & Richardson, P. (2010). The role of affect in the estimation of risk. *Journal of Mental Health, 19*(5), 444–451.

Further reading

A classic text by a Nobel Prize winner looking at risk judgements from a behavioural economics perspective – a little dense at times, but a fascinating insight into highly relevant cognitive errors that we all make in judging risk.

Kahneman, D. (2011). Thinking, Fast and Slow. UK: Allen Lane.

There are numerous books written on the subject of risk assessment and offending behaviour.

For violent offending risk assessment:

Webster, C., Haque, Q., & Hucker, S. (2013) Violence Risk-Assessment and Management: Advances Through Structured Professional Judgement and Sequential Redirections. Chichester: John Wiley & Sons Ltd.

For sexual offending risk assessment:

Craissati, J. (2019) The Rehabilitation of Sexual Offenders: Complexity, Risk and Desistance. London: Routledge.

Taking a slightly different approach, incorporating psychodynamic ideas:

Blumenthal, S., Wood, H., & Williams, A. (2018). Assessing Risk: A Relational Approach. London: Routledge.

7 Owen's story

Personality disorder and psychopathy: mad or bad?

Understanding personality disorder in a meaningful way

Personality disorder is an unpleasant term, with connotations of personal defectiveness and stigmatising labelling; furthermore, within mental health and criminal justice services, the diagnosis – for that is what it is – is known to be associated with a greater likelihood of exclusion from services. In other words, from the individual's perspective, to be personality disordered means that one may not be worthy of mental health support, and that behaviour associated with the diagnosis is deemed 'bad not mad' and therefore not requiring empathy or compassion.

The reader may wonder why the term has persisted to the present day if it is associated with such negativity. The condensed answer – at least when working with individuals who have committed serious offences – is that research clearly shows us that personality disorder matters. It matters because it is associated with worse outcomes, for men who offend, in a variety of ways: higher levels of sexual and physically violent reoffending, higher levels of failure to engage in and complete treatment, higher levels of non-compliance with community requirements, and a return to prison. Personality disorder is also associated with institutional and organisational disruption: greater numbers of spurious complaints, poor staff behaviour and staff burnout in response to behaviours that are challenging, and high levels of self-harm and therefore also a risk of suicide in the offenders; individuals with the label often misuse substances, and are more likely to die young by means of accidental overdoses and other impulsive or reckless acts that endangers their and others' lives.

This chapter therefore aims to set out a straightforward and simple model for understanding the underlying psychological principles associated with the term personality disorder. It is actually the case that the majority of case vignettes detailed in this book would have been described as personality disordered at the time of their trial. As we have followed their bumpy pathways through the prison system, there are indications that the traits causing the individuals their most striking problems – the impasse and negativity they encounter, the self-destructive behaviours – can be attributed to those persistent psychological features of their personality. However, thus far, the diagnosis was not emphasised as it added little or nothing of value to the narrative. The reader will make their own decision at the end of this chapter as to whether the label adds substantially to our understanding of complex individuals with serious offending histories.

The prevalence and nature of personality disorder

Numerous studies that use structured approaches to identifying personality disorder in the general population have arrived at similar conclusions: it comprises about 10% of all those going to the GP (primary care), 25% of those with an admission to psychiatric hospital (secondary care), and about 60% of those in prison. We might conclude that the label is of diminishing utility as its prevalence rises, either for those who receive it or those who bestow it. In particular, of the 60% of prisoners who meet the diagnostic criteria for personality disorder, around 80% are labelled 'antisocial' (sometimes referred to as 'dissocial'). This seems rather ridiculous and unhelpful, frankly, and we might reasonably conclude that these diagnostic criteria are socially driven and overly reliant on 'bad behaviour' as a definition.

A further difficulty with the label is the idea of a diagnosis based on simple presence or absence of symptoms; this approach works better for physical problems such as an infection or a broken limb – one either has it or one does not. However, for complex issues such as personality difficulties, current approaches emphasise the undoubted benefits of considering the problem as lying on a continuum: that is, personality traits can be highly functional, moderately problematic, or severely disruptive to the individual and his/her network and community.

Box 7.1 outlines a continuum-based approach to personality difficulties that does not rely on a diagnosis, and addresses myths regarding prognosis and treatability. In this simple model, personality difficulties are conceptualised as falling along a continuum of severity and covering three essential domains. The 'three P's' require personality traits and behaviours to

BOX 7.1

Defining personality disorder: the three P's

PROBLEMATIC

Traits are considered to be abnormal (outside the normal range for the culture and society in which they are observed).

PERVASIVE

Traits or symptoms appear in several domains of functioning; for example, as emotional difficulties, problems in thinking styles, behavioural issues, and problematic ways of relating to others.

PERSISTENT

Traits or symptoms emerge in late adolescence or early adulthood usually and persist over many years.

- Core traits (such as emotional sensitivity, callousness, or suspiciousness) tend to be largely impervious to the effects of maturation or therapeutic interventions and remain indefinitely.
- Secondary behavioural traits (such as self-harm, excessive substance misuse, violent outbursts, harassing behaviours, or frequent failures in employment or relationships) tend to improve with maturity or in response to therapeutic interventions, albeit more slowly than for the average person.

Note: Applying the principle of the three P's means that a person cannot be thought to have a personality disorder on the basis of their offending behaviour alone.

be problematic, pervasive, and persistent. Furthermore, we now know that a diagnosis of personality disorder is no longer the lifelong label – resistant to all forms of treatment – that professionals used to believe. Box 7.1 details how problematic characteristics can fall into two broad categories: those that are core to the individual, quite possibly biological in origin, and persistent; and those that are more behaviourally focused and responsive to maturation and therapeutic interventions, a sort of 'mellowing with age' that we can all observe in ourselves and our loved ones, as well as in the examples in this book. Research studies that have followed up individuals with diagnoses of either emotionally unstable (borderline) or antisocial (dissocial) personality disorder over a ten-year period, have found that around 80% no longer meet diagnostic criteria, even though they may continue to experience difficulties at particularly challenging periods in their life.[1]

In order to bring the three P's approach to life, it is helpful to consider two labels – narcissistic and paranoid – that can be associated with personality difficulties, but with which the general public are also reasonably conversant. If we take the label narcissistic, then we might commonly see such traits in small doses in strong leaders and successful businessmen; these may be individuals characterised by self-confidence and absence of doubt, who engage in assertive and charismatic interactions with others. In moderate doses, perhaps noticeable at work, narcissistic individuals might struggle to work in teams, and be seen as overly competitive by work peers, and highly sensitive to criticism, responding badly to feedback; but at home, with a partner who has a soothing manner and is keen to take the role of homemaker, life might proceed more harmoniously. However, for those with narcissistic traits that dominate their interactions with the world in all spheres of life, these characteristics are more likely ultimately to be self-destructive, causing distress to others, and difficulties for the individual him/herself. We will learn more about this when considering psychopathy later in the chapter.

We can take the same approach to the label 'paranoid' – a trait most people would understand as associated with suspiciousness regarding the motives of others and a propensity to consider the actions of others as potentially malign. In small doses, such individuals might be appropriately cautious when signing documents, or interpreting media reports, weighing up information with a healthy degree of scepticism, more so than family or friends. In moderate doses, individuals with paranoid traits might be seen as eccentric individuals with peculiar or unusual beliefs in certain conspiracy theories, otherwise leading their lives in fairly ordinary ways; avoid that particular topic of conversation, and nothing untoward would be noted. However, for those who experience every interaction with others as a potential threat, constant vigilance and hostile accusations alienate everyone around them, and can lead to problems with accusations of harassment/stalking/aggressive threats in response to situations that the average person might find unremarkable.

Personality difficulties and trauma: understanding the bio-psycho-social model

Personality development provides a useful focus for the nature-nurture debate, as the literature has lurched from historical ideas of trauma and disturbed attachment to more contemporary research into biological imperatives underpinning personality. The truth seems to lie somewhere in-between these two polar positions: our personalities are surprisingly influenced by our genetic and biological predispositions – probably accounting for around 40% of personality variation – and our early familial and social environments interact with these underlying temperaments in order to determine the developing shape of an individual's personality and interactions with the world around them. The narratives in this book have been strongly driven by these early interactions that influence the various pathways into serious crimes of violence. Therefore, when we consider those who shatter the lives of others and whose own lives are also shattered as a result of violent acts, we tend to think of personality difficulties in terms of the bio-psycho-social model. Known biological predispositions include callous and unemotional traits, cognitive rigidity, emotional sensitivity, and aggressiveness, although these are probably not the only genetically driven traits. There is, however, no gene for paranoid or narcissistic personality. The biological predispositions interact with the individual's experience of attachment to primary carers within the familial environment (see Chapter 2) and/or with childhood experiences of complex trauma (see Chapter 5) to shape personality. Psychologists tend to underestimate the influence of social factors in shaping the individual, but this is a mistake; not only are there significant cultural and social variations in what is considered abnormal behaviour, but there are varying social norms that drive the expression of distress. For example, it is generally thought that societies viewed from an eastern perspective emphasise the importance of community and de-emphasise the importance of the individual; these cultures tend to result in personality difficulties that are more inward focused and self-blaming. Conversely, viewed from a western perspective, societies tend to emphasise the individual over community, and personality difficulties are more commonly externally focused and associated with behaviours that have an impact on the environment. Other factors such as socio-economic status (including poverty and lack of financial opportunities), social experiences such as exposure to racist attitudes, or social influences such as exclusive exposure to an antisocial peer group may all aggravate underlying vulnerabilities in relation to personality difficulties.

As a brief example of this model, consider Nick – someone who acquired a label of paranoid and antisocial personality disorder. Nick is an individual with a rather rigid cognitive style and poor reality testing (bio) by which we mean that he tends to engage in very black and white thinking and is poor at 'horizon-scanning' for breadth of meaning in the world around him. He also repeatedly witnessed the domestic abuse of his mother by his father, and experienced this as intensely frightening, with the result that this led to a rather hyper-vigilant approach to considering men as a potential threat to him (psycho). In his wider community – a socially deprived and often lawless urban environment – Nick was exposed to only one type of male authority that could provide an alternative model of what it means to be a man, his antisocial peers. However, these peers are also those who can threaten his rather fragile sense of himself as strong and invulnerable (social). He had to maintain vigilance in response to these threats – it led to violence in terms of his hypersensitivity to perceived humiliation in everyday interactions with his peers that others might view as probably benign. For example, innocuous arguments between Nick and associates might escalate to violence when interpreted by him as attempts to challenge his standing in the eyes of others. This personality style of Nick's was problematic not only in relation to his history of offending, but was also present in his response in prison to those – usually prison officers – who were in authority; and it was noticeable within his intimate relationships in which he showed particularly controlling and 'paranoid' behaviours.

Applying the bio-psycho-social model to an understanding of psychopathy

No chapter on personality and its association with violent crime can be concluded without reference to the concept of psychopathy. Again, this is a term that is in the public domain and associated with ideas of dangerousness – even serial killing, lack of empathy, and unpredictability (akin to ideas of not being quite like others). Although not a formal subtype of personality diagnosis in the diagnostic manuals for mental disorder like the terms narcissistic and paranoid, it is nevertheless a problematic personality type, characterised by the 3 P's, associated with negative outcomes in those who have offending backgrounds, and considered extremely challenging to manage or to treat therapeutically. Psychopathy also holds the same level of controversy within the relevant professional groups as the broader term, personality disorder, although no one argues that it is entirely spurious or fictitious as a 'type'.

The concept of psychopathy has been widely studied; it is found in around 1% of the general male population, in 8% of the male prisoner population, and in 2% of the female prison population. Rates are slightly higher in North America for reasons that are not entirely clear. A seminal early text on psychopathy was *The Mask of Sanity* (Cleckley, 1941), in which Cleckley emphasised the fake quality of apparent normal human interactions in the psychopath that represented a mask, obscuring the inability of the individual

BOX 7.2

The four facets of the Psychopathy Checklist

Factor 1: Interpersonal/affective

- ***Facet 1: Interpersonal***
  These are traits that indicate a strong propensity for superficial charm and arrogance in terms of personality, with behaviours that include excessive lying to others and conning or manipulative behaviours.
- ***Facet 2: Affective***
  Emotional responses in a variety of situations that suggest a lack of feelings of guilt, shallow or fake emotions, callousness, and difficulty in taking personal responsibility for behaviour.

Factor 2: Social deviance

- ***Facet 3: Lifestyle***
  Behaviours that indicate a strong tendency towards boredom associated with repeatedly impulsive and irresponsible behaviours. This includes a propensity to exploit others for financial support and holding unrealistic longer term goals.
- ***Facet 4: Antisocial***
  Behaviours that are largely historical, including child, adolescent, and adult problems with rule breaking – including repeated, serious, and/or diverse offending.

to experience emotions as others might. Practitioners in the field will now automatically think of the Psychopathy Checklist (Hare, 1991) as the more contemporary approach to assessing the nature of the psychopathic individual; and this checklist introduces a range of behavioural concerns as well as the core personality features identified by Cleckley. The Psychopathy Checklist (PCL-R) comprises 20 items that define the psychopath in fairly objective and standardised terms, and we return to this later in the chapter, with the traits being detailed in Box 7.2.

If we return to the bio-psycho-social model, this also applies to psychopathy, although there is probably more evidence for the biological component in the make-up of the psychopathic individual. There are numerous brain studies of individuals assessed as having psychopathic traits, and also immensely interesting – albeit controversial and morally uncomfortable – primate studies. Famous studies of chimpanzees, who were either reared with their mothers (competent and caring) or in a nursery environment (having had failing or ill mothers), examined genetic traits and behaviours associated with psychopathy. It was found that there were broadly three relevant genetic elements that led to observed behaviours that were strongly biologically determined regardless of the rearing experience (although it should be noted that rearing experience provided some added complexities to the situation that would support an element of environmental influence on behaviour). The genetically driven features were *disinhibition* (difficulty delaying gratification), *meanness* (callous and unemotional traits), and *boldness* (characterised by a greater number of fearless or dominant behaviours). It was found that those chimpanzees who demonstrated biological drivers for disinhibition and meanness were significantly more likely to engage in *callous aggression*.

In terms of human studies, the two biological correlates most commonly cited in terms of brain function in psychopathy are abnormalities in those areas of the brain responsible for emotional processing and learning, and moral decision-making. To explain further:

- ***Emotional processing***
  Brain and behaviour research shows that an attack stops once one of the participants displays submission cues – such as a sad facial expression or tears – and this assists with the development of empathy and remorse, which in turn promote pro-social behaviours and stronger social bonds. This mechanism is significantly impaired in individuals with psychopathic features; whilst such individuals are as good at recognising others' emotions as the wider population, they fail to become emotionally engaged and so do not appear to have the capacity to feel for others. This underpins the observation that psychopathic individuals have shallow and/or fake emotions, and appear to be adept at manipulating others to their own ends.
- ***Moral decision-making***
  When making a decision, individuals with psychopathic traits are more insensitive to the negative consequences ensuing from their choices; in other words, decision-making processes are not mediated by emotional responses that have embedded as a result of learning from previous mistakes. It is this element of the personality difficulties that can be so destructive or disabling for the psychopathic individual as s/he fails to adapt their response to the world or to control their behaviour in the light of learning experiences.

Box 7.2 outlines the key elements of the Psychopathy Checklist (PCL-R), clustering the items around the two factors and four facets that make up the assessment. With a possible total score of 40, it is actually quite difficult to score over 30 (the commonly used cut-off point for psychopathy); but different combinations of scores imply that there is no one 'type' of psychopath. It is possible, for example, to be emotionally and behaviourally volatile and a psychopath, or a cold and calculating psychopath; to be very noticeably narcissistic and vicious but self-controlled, or to be highly impulsive and antisocial with limited empathy for others. Killing – let alone more than one killing – is not a prerequisite as a range of multiple minor offences might suffice to meet the 'antisocial' criteria. It may conceivably be possible for a politician to meet the criteria – a popular but unsubstantiated assertion – but only if there is clear evidence for most of the antisocial behaviours as well as the personal characteristics of callousness and ruthlessness.

The reader will now have a reasonably good understanding of the basic concepts that drive our understanding of personality as applied to the world of serious violent offending. However, it feels rather abstract and theoretical until applied to real people facing real-life choices. The rest of this chapter is devoted to Owen and his narrative regarding the pathway into offending, but most particularly, focusing on his traits and behaviours that ultimately gave rise to the conclusion that he was struggling with very marked psychopathic traits. The reader may wish to consider how Owen demonstrated the 3 P's – as described in Box 7.1 – and met criteria for psychopathy – as described in Box 7.2.

Owen's story

I first met Owen when he was in high secure prison, serving a life sentence for murder; he had already spent 29 years in prison of which the first 14 were spent serving his tariff (the punishment period) and a further 15 years had passed during which time his attempts to progress via Parole Board hearings had met with variable success. Ten years previously, he had progressed as far as open prison, where he failed to return from a town visit until the next day – for no justifiable reason – and had been returned to closed prison. He had then been assessed for psychopathy by a concerned prison psychology department and found to reach the threshold; a specialist programme of interventions was recommended, but Owen dug his heels in, vigorously challenged the psychopathy assessment via quasi-legal means, and refused to speak to psychologists or to participate in his sentence plan. It took several years – associated with the gradual maturation that has often played a part in the progress of the individuals described in this book – and a good solicitor, before Owen was sufficiently mellow and receptive to agree to an independent psychology assessment. My task was to identify a more psychologically attuned approach to his management – ideally engaging him in the process – that might break the impasse. As someone outside the prison service, I was fortunate in not being tainted by the *'duplicitous nature of authority'* in the prison staff, as he viewed it.

Before sharing the details of Owen's narrative about his pathway into prison, it may be helpful to pause and consider the impact of his presence on the interviewer. It is sometimes said that one can discern the presence of psychopathy by noticing the emotional response that the individual provokes in oneself when interacting; indeed, fictitious media portrayals support this idea when they emphasise the icy charm with which the psychopath traps his prey. The reality is rather more mundane, and although it is crucial to test the tone and impression of the practitioner-offender interaction, the predictive reliability of the therapist-client relationship is variable. As is quite often the case, Owen provoked in me two quite contrasting emotions, and I vacillated between the two in a confused manner throughout our time together. There is no doubt that he could be immensely likeable, not because of his superficial charm which he could turn on if he wished – and for the most part he did not wish to when I saw him! However, I liked his engaging and lively mind, driven by an intelligence that meant he was quick witted and considered the world around him with a sharp perceptiveness that could, admittedly, also be a weapon – humiliating or dismissing staff with a contemptuous retort. This intelligence was coupled with a searing honesty in relation to matters about which other prisoners knew they ought to dissemble; for example, he was unabashedly but refreshingly frank in admitting his callousness in relation to others, it simply did not matter to him what other people thought about this aspect of his nature. On the other hand, he could be absolutely infuriating, arguing every point with pedantry; choosing, for example, to waste the time allotted for him to see me by arguing with prison officers as to whether he had to wear a prison shirt for the interview, such that I had to rearrange the appointment. His honesty could also be cruel, particularly if he was annoyed, and at such times, one had a glimpse of the man who had killed when thwarted.

Owen had always said that he was *'the black sheep of the family'*. He was the third of four children, with hard-working and caring parents; no one had a criminal record or mental health difficulties, and his siblings had all progressed reasonably well at school and were settled with jobs and families in adulthood. It is the case that his parents separated and then divorced when he was aged around 11, but their unhappiness together did not spill over into issues of emotional neglect or physical abuse within the family. In other words, it was not possible to identify early family issues that might have driven Owen's subsequent pathway. Owen did, however, have a stutter when he was young, and was late to develop clear and fluent speech, which led to some bullying of him at primary school; he denied any significant emotional impact of this experience but agreed that it made him fiercely determined to overcome the problem and never again to allow himself to be humiliated or made vulnerable by any visible weakness.

Behavioural problems were reported by the school and by his parents from an early age, and the latter were being asked to attend primary school to deal with Owen's disruptive behaviour, ultimately leading to a number of brief suspensions. Owen's explanation, looking back, was simply that '*it was more exciting*' (to behave badly). At secondary school he was considered to be bright, but his behaviour meant that he was kept down a year about which he felt intensely aggrieved '*because I was far too bright for the others, I should have been a year ahead, not behind*'. By the age of 12, Owen was in trouble with the police for a series of relatively minor offences such as criminal damage (throwing milk bottles at front doors), theft (stealing from back gardens and shops), and burglary (stealing metal scrap from building sites). By the age of 15, he was the most notorious of a group of delinquent boys who all lived locally, truanting from school, and organising themselves into unofficial gangs with the primary aim of making pocket money by dealing drugs. Owen insisted – probably with some truth to it – that his experience of being falsely accused (as he maintained it) by the police of armed robbery at the age of 18 was a turning point for him. Of course, this accusation may not have been false, as Owen was quite capable of playing mischievously with his own life story to suit his own ends; however, his account was that he was enraged by the authorities' manipulation of the truth in relation to this offence, that he was '*fitted up*', and his offer of a place at university was '*scuppered*'; finally, 11 months on remand at a young offenders prison '*sealed my fate … I knew then that I had nothing to lose, I was determined to show everyone what kind of criminal I could be – a successful one, someone who could pull one over on the police*'. At first, this reasoning seems faulty, somewhat perplexing; but it is important to understand that for Owen, he experienced the false accusation as an intensely personal attack on his integrity, and something that he viewed as thwarting his aspirations – however unrealistic – to be someone of academic standing and ability. This brooding resentment was nurtured by him and transformed into an entitled and vengeful state of mind against authority – '*I felt justified in taking from others, because I was owed it*'. From that point on, Owen's offending was prolific, although he was arrested relatively rarely. Nevertheless, in early adulthood, he was convicted of a series of robberies and possession of weapons (a knife and then an imitation firearm) and by the time he was 32 – when he committed the offence for which he was serving a life sentence – he had spent much of his adult life either in prison or living a moderately *'flashy'* lifestyle off the proceeds of crack cocaine and heroin sales.

Despite time in prison and drug dealing, Owen had held a few short-term jobs, but was quickly bored or was sacked for unreliability. His longest period of employment had been as a nightclub bouncer; Owen liked to describe the ways in which he learnt to provoke aggressive reactions in customers that would then provide the excuse he needed to use physical violence to control them. In terms of relationships, he had had a string of sexual encounters from mid-adolescence onwards. There was a suggestion that he had been hurt by a girlfriend's rejection early on, although he did not like to talk about this; however, he spoke openly and unapologetically about his promiscuity, saying that *'it's best to have two or three on the go, rather than one that can leave me'*. He cited two women as influential insofar as they were the mothers of his children – one daughter and one son – and each of these relationships had endured several months, although he had been persistently unfaithful throughout and had made no financial provision for his children. Owen had never seen his daughter, but he had kept in touch with his son's mother, and had had telephone contact with his son during his prison sentence. Although his behaviour would suggest he was largely indifferent in his feelings towards his daughter, he was undoubtedly drawn to have a connection with his son, seeing him somewhat as a reflection or extension of himself of which he could then feel proud.

The index offence was shockingly violent, but in other ways perhaps unremarkable. Owen and various co-defendants were engaged in a number of street robberies, using the proceeds variably to trade crack cocaine or to consume large quantities of the drug themselves. The victim – a postman – was the last in a successful string of robberies, a man who simply resisted the snatching of his wallet and postal bag. On this occasion, Owen was operating alone, and he was enraged by the victim's resistance, persisted with the robbery and lashed out at the man, knocking the victim to the ground and then embarking on an appallingly vicious attack, kicking and jumping on the victim's head, and leaving him for dead. In fact, the victim was not dead, but dreadfully injured; he was treated in hospital for several months before dying of a hospital-acquired infection. Charged with murder, Owen admitted to the robbery and to grievous bodily harm, but maintained – and continued to maintain for the next 29 years – that he could not be made responsible for the victim's death, which *'wasn't my fault'*. Interestingly, in another person with a different personality style, it seemed to me it would have been possible to engage in a more reflective and empathic discussion about the ways in which feelings of shame and regret interfered with the perpetrator's ability to think clearly about the unintended consequences of his/her loss of control. However, Owen did not feel any shame – or such feelings were so buried they were inaccessible – and therefore any debate regarding moral responsibility and understanding the consequences of behaviour was experienced by Owen as illogical and patronising; this often led to an unhelpful standoff with professionals who experienced the vacuum of empathy as abhorrent, and who became particularly hostile to his stance as a result.

In prison, Owen continued to subvert and provoke the system, initially in overtly violent ways, and then over time by more subtle and less deliberate means. For example, the number of fights with staff and other prisoners reduced over time, as did weeks spent in the Segregation Unit; he went from brewing hooch (illegal alcohol) and being known as a gang leader on the wing, to someone who was suspected of stirring unrest and trading in illegal goods, but who more often managed to stay under the radar of the authorities. There were also some concerns regarding his interactions with female staff: 15 years previously a female prison officer had been sacked for bringing in a mobile phone for him, and 5 years previously he had had an affair with his prison visitor; she was then barred entry to the prison when this was found out, and not able to work as a visitor anymore. However, Owen kept the relationship going, openly acknowledging that although he '*quite liked her*', his primary motive was to ensure that he had a supply of visits, money, and other useful items.

Despite the mellowing of his attitude and behaviour with time and age, there continued to be numerous intelligence reports about him; these are snippets of information/concerns that are conveyed by staff or by prisoners to the security department of a prison, and that are ranked for reliability. Intelligence reports – although often malicious and unreliable – could be thought of as a reasonably good barometer of the extent to which a prisoner's personality is problematic within the institution. Suspicions that Owen was dealing drugs within the prison in recent years were found to be false – he was buying and selling legal goods on behalf of other prisoners, with the assistance of his girlfriend (the former prison visitor) – and thereby running a small but profitable '*legal*' business. Nevertheless, Owen's negative reputation was long-standing, and few staff truly believed that his activity was legitimate. Reports to the Parole Board were persistently negative, particular due to the litany of historical concerns, and partly because Owen was so uncompromising in his attitude and behaviour, persistently belittling the regime and its staff, and refusing to participate in more therapeutic interventions.

Understanding and managing Owen's psychopathic traits

Pausing for a moment, it is helpful to review Owen's narrative against the description of traits and behaviours contained in the Psychopathy Checklist, as summarised in Box 7.2, in order to understand why he might have scored high on such a personality tool. If we consider the *interpersonal facet*, then there is considerable evidence for many of the items relating to glib and superficial relationships and behaviours that manipulate others to meet his own needs; however, there is no evidence for really problematic lying as he was much more prone to excessive honesty when it suited him. Similarly, for the *affective (emotional) facet*, there is a strong sense of his shallow emotional state, his capacity for chilling callousness, and his stubborn inability to take responsibility for his actions. The *lifestyle facet* is strongly present in terms of a propensity for boredom and seeking excitement which is a strong thread throughout his life, and there is a good deal of evidence for using others for financial gain. However, there is room for uncertainty in relation to impulsivity as he presents with a mixed picture of highly controlling and poorly controlled behaviours, and there are some doubts as to whether all his goals are unrealistic or simply difficult to attain. Finally, the *antisocial facet* – relying as it does on historical facts to a great extent – undoubtedly points to an individual who demonstrated problematic behaviours from an unusually early age, particularly in terms of arrests before the age of 13. For so many prisoners, this could be understood in terms of family and social adversity, but interestingly in Owen's case, although there are developmental factors – such as his stutter – that shaped his experience of the world, these cannot on their own account for the subsequent pathway into unusually prolonged and destructive behaviours. The absence of adversity in the home environment does point to the likely salience of biological factors driving his early behaviours.

At this point, do we give up all hope for Owen and his capacity for rehabilitation? The only question for professionals and for the Parole Board is whether he will persist in posing a risk of further significant violence to others because a decision to release can only be granted if the risk is thought to be low and the risk management plan strong. In order to answer that question, we need to know which of his traits are most closely linked to risk of violence and which might be amenable to change. As with all pervasive personality problems – clearly described in Box 7.1 – we need to differentiate between core, immutable characteristics, and secondary changeable behaviours. In the case of psychopathy, it is Factor 1 characteristics that barely change over time, but tend only to be linked to problems with management rather than risk to others; Factor 2 elements – the antisocial features – are the most closely related to risk to others, but are indicative of the behavioural characteristics that most respond to maturation and interventions.

Owen's story, to my mind, provides a very clear picture of someone who remains as provocative, frustrating, and callous as the day he committed the index offence, but whose decisions and behaviour have increasingly shown an amelioration in key risk concerns. Approaches by professionals that understandably focused on his deficits – too much bad behaviour and too little appropriate emotion – were met by him with implacable opposition. Approaches that adopted a stance of promoting 'enlightened self-interest' were the most successful, but these required the ability of the professional to manage their own impulses to put Owen in his place! Enlightened self-interest is an approach taken for individuals who have very marked features of narcissistic and/or psychopathic personality traits; it involves identifying features that are problematic when driving antisocial behaviours, but which can be redirected as a strength in achieving pro-social goals. For example, it was immensely tempting to point out to Owen – despite knowing that it would result in impasse – the reality that his supremely self-confident and arrogant statements regarding his academic ability were doubtful, that he had lied about his university place in his late teens, and that he did not have GCSE maths or English. In contrast, taking an enlightened self-interest approach, a visiting teacher went out of his way to secure some charitable funding for Owen to pursue open university qualifications – despite the irritation of staff who felt he was receiving undeserved special treatment – and the number of disruptive behaviours and repeated formal complaints he submitted reduced significantly. Similarly, once Owen was given a scoring sheet for the PCL-R and undertook his own assessment in discussion with me in interview, he was interested despite himself, and curious to '*see how I score*'; we ended up cordially agreeing to differ in our scoring by only one point! Of course, Owen still exaggerated his academic progress if asked, but by encouraging staff to withhold comment and thereby humiliation, he became less sensitive about perceived slights. Improved behaviour led to Owen being offered a valued prison job by an enlightened senior prison officer, and so, step by step, his previous difficulties – risk taking, controlling behaviour, arrogance and so on – were channelled into pro-social goals; disruptive behaviour converted into formal complaints, and a refusal to comply with orders converted into an assertive (sometimes too much so) approach to arguing his point of view.

Conclusion: taking a cautiously hopeful stance to rehabilitation

Eventually, Owen was released by the Parole Board, after several false starts and a good deal of understandable nervousness. Despite 30 years in prison, his intelligence and wit remained as sharp as ever, and there was no deterioration in his coping skills suggestive of institutionalisation. He quietly extricated himself from the expectations of his girlfriend, and managed all resettlement tasks without faltering; in his charming and compelling way, he managed to persuade a criminal justice charity to take him on as a volunteer, and he thoroughly enjoyed his new role as a reformed offender educating those at risk of a life of crime. One year after his release, Owen found himself in serious trouble when some money went missing from the charity's petty cash – money that Owen had *'borrowed'* to help out a former prisoner acquaintance of his who was in trouble. There was considerable pressure on the probation service to recall Owen to prison, on the basis that here was evidence of the duplicitous nature of his personality, his leaning towards antisocial behaviour, and the first sight of a slippery slope into violence. He was not assisted by his past reputation, or his current propensity to make numerous rather entitled complaints regarding the probation service and the inadequacy of their service offer as he viewed it. However, Owen's return to prison was a relatively brief one of around nine months: the charity did indeed confirm eventually that Owen had told a work colleague of his intention to take but then repay the money. Although his actions were strictly illegal and he would not be allowed to return to the charity, the Parole Board agreed that it was complacency and a habitual pattern of rewriting the rules to suit himself that had led to problems; they were satisfied that no acts of violence had occurred for 12 years in prison and 1 year in the community, and that there was only a very tenuous link between the incident and future violence. The return to prison had been a salutary lesson for him; although Owen stood by his motives for the incident in his usual stubborn and defensive way, he was willing to concede that his decision-making had been ill thought out. There were tentative signs of an emotional response when Owen talked about *'letting my son down'* as he had begun to forge something of a relationship with his adult son, and felt embarrassed to explain that he was back in prison. Critics of Owen pointed out that his feelings for his son were entirely self-interested, and not a sign of a strong emotional bond; this was possibly true, but not actually relevant to the likely success of his rerelease. The fact is that academic attainment and a connection to his son were strong pro-social motivators for Owen, regardless of their superficiality or links to his profound arrogance. Whether Owen will manage to sustain a crime-free life in the community is uncertain, although it seems increasingly likely that he will manage to remain violence-free. The question for all of us is whether the identification of psychopathy significantly added to the quality and likely success of the risk management approach for Owen, or whether it imposed a tremendously stigmatising label on him that aggravated the negative reactions experienced by all who were tasked with his management.

Note

1. For example, Skodol, A.E., Gunderson, J.G., Shea, M.T. et al. (2005) The Collaborative Longitudinal Personality Disorders Study (CLPS): overview and implications. *Journal of Personality Disorders.* , 19 (5), 487–504.

Further reading

There are numerous academic texts written about both personality disorder and psychopathy. For the interested reader, Cleckley's book remains a seminal text. With the considerable developments now in the United Kingdom to services for individuals with personality difficulties and offending behaviour, there is a highly accessible Practitioner Guide available free to download. This targets non-specialist staff working in public and voluntary sector organisations and is full of tips and case vignettes that bring the subject to life.

Cleckley, H. (1941). *The Mask of Sanity*. Various publishers, according to different editions.

HMPPS and NHS (2019). Practitioner Guide: Working with People in the Criminal Justice System Showing Personality Difficulties. https://assets.publishing.service.gov.uk/government/uploads/system/uploads/attachment_data/file/869843/6.5151_HMPPS_Working_with_Offenders_with_Personality_Disorder_v17_WEB.pdf

For further – but rather technical – information on the primate studies, read the following and related articles:

Latzman, R., Schapiro, S., & Hopkins, W. (2017) Triarchic psychopathy dimensions in chimpanzees (*Pan troglodytes*): investigating associations with genetic variation in the vasopressin receptor 1A gene. *Frontiers in Neuroscience, 11*, 407.

For a relatively accessible systematic review of the published literature on the link between personality disorder and violence:

Lowenstein, J., Purvis, C., & Rose, K. (2016). A systematic review on the relationship between antisocial, borderline and narcissistic personality disorder diagnostic traits and risk of violence to others in a clinical and forensic sample. *Borderline Personality Disorder and Emotion Dysregulation, 3*, 14.

8

Peter, Quinn, Rob, and Stuart's story

Severe mental illness and violence: understanding risk and responsibility for those who are violent

> 'An inquiry has been commissioned after a man with paranoid schizophrenia who had lost touch with mental health services killed a stranger in a holiday town with a throwing knife.'
>
> 'M***, who has paranoid schizophrenia, was jailed for life for murdering C*** on a train. … He killed C*** by stabbing him 18 times in 25 seconds in front of his 14-year-old son. A psychiatrist had deemed him to be no threat to himself or others the day before the attack.'
>
> 'A paranoid schizophrenic, who killed three pensioners in the space of a few hours in Exeter, has been found not guilty of murder by reason of insanity. … (He) was suffering from delusions that led him to wrongly believe he was uncovering a paedophile ring, his trial heard.'

This is the first page of the search engine when typing in 'psychiatric patient kills 2019', three terrible tragedies reported by UK national newspapers; note the themes of frenzied knife use, terrifyingly unexpected attacks that intrude on the victim's everyday life, and the implication that mental health services had failed in some way.

This chapter is about severe mental illness and its association with violence, exploring whether the above media reporting reflects a painful reality about the nature of the illness or is promoting myths about the nature of madness – demonising people whose 'otherness' is alien to us and therefore frightening. To explore this issue, the topic needs to be simplified (see Box 8.1) as the diagnosis and understanding of severe mental illness is not without uncertainty, complexity, and controversy. There is a good deal of research on the topic of illness and violence, and a summary of the facts about the link with violence is laid out in Box 8.2. However, it is the four case stories – Peter, Quinn, Rob, and Stuart – that bring to life the way in which severe mental illness may link to acts of serious violence.

BOX 8.1

Definitions of psychosis and its symptoms

PSYCHOSIS

A state in which a person perceives or interprets reality in a very different way from the people around them, such that s/he could be described as having 'lost touch with reality'.

THE MAIN SYMPTOMS OF PSYCHOSIS

Hallucinations

A sensory perception in the absence of stimuli. Most commonly this takes the form of hearing voices (when there is no one actually speaking to the person) that are perceived to be emanating from outside the person's head that talk to them or about them – and sometimes command them to do things. However, hallucinations can be experienced in all five senses; for example, older adults with an infection-induced psychosis might report visual hallucinations.

Delusions

A sustained belief that nobody shares and which other experiences or perceptions show cannot be true, although it feels very real to the person him/herself. These 'false beliefs' can be persecutory in nature; that is, when a person believes that someone or something is attempting to harm them.

Disorganised thinking and speech

Characteristics might include racing thoughts leading to stumbling over words, rapidly switching topics, or switching to topics that are unrelated, incomprehensible speech in which words are linked because of the way they sound, for example, rather than for their meaning.

NEGATIVE SYMPTOMS

These symptoms tend to have an impact on an individual's personality and interpersonal functioning, and may endure long after the 'positive symptoms' – described above – have ameliorated. Such symptoms describe deficits states (or a 'lack of') in an individual, including

- Reduced emotional expression
- Decreased motivation and apathy
- A lack of interest
- Social withdrawal
- Reduced spontaneous speech

What is severe mental illness?

Mental illness, mental disorder, severe illness, schizophrenia, manic depression, bipolar disorder, borderline personality.... The reader may well be understandably confused as to whether these are distinct or overlapping terms; the answer is that they are often used interchangeably, even by professionals. It is much easier for us to focus on the term psychosis for the purposes of this chapter (see Box 8.1 for all the definitions of terms). Psychosis is the term for when a person loses touch with reality, and it can be thought of as a single episode, an enduring or an intermittent state of mind. There are a number of medical conditions that can trigger a psychosis: it could be an illness such as schizophrenia or bipolar disorder (previously known as manic depression) or a very severe depression; excessive sleep deprivation, reactions to medications, and toxic states of infection can all trigger psychosis; and then psychosis can also be triggered by alcohol or illicit drug misuse or after women have given birth. The symptoms of psychosis that the general public might be most familiar with are hallucinations and delusions; these are 'false' sensory experiences and beliefs whose content is strongly influenced by cultural norms and regional differences, as well as fluctuating in theme across time. For example, it used to be more common that individuals with a psychotic disorder experienced visual hallucinations (seeing things) primarily, but now it is auditory hallucinations (hearing voices) that predominate; delusional beliefs of a persecutory nature in the United Kingdom used to be linked to the secret service or the IRA, but are now more likely to reflect themes of Islamic extremism or paedophilia – social concerns that are repeatedly highlighted in the media. Determining whether or not an auditory hallucination or delusional belief is linked to a psychotic episode (or mental illness) is not entirely straightforward: many individuals in the general population report hearing voices, and this is a particularly common phenomenon with the recently bereaved. False beliefs can also be difficult to determine in all cases, as otherwise stable and ordinary individuals can report extremely unusual and firmly held beliefs – for example, relating to alien abduction – that most of us would tend to reject as impossible. Nevertheless, such individuals may not be mentally ill.

The less well-known symptoms of psychosis relate to thought disorder – disorganised thinking and speech – symptoms that indicate a more fragmented state of mind. Perhaps the more neglected consequences of a psychotic illness in the public's awareness are the negative symptoms that can emerge, as these have such a debilitating impact on the sufferer's social functioning and integration with society.

The causes of psychosis

Here we return to the nature-nurture debate that we encountered when discussing the development of personality difficulties. To circumvent the controversies in this debate about the causes of mental illness, it is probably most helpful to focus on the stress-vulnerability model of psychosis, particularly as it pertains to an underlying illness such as schizophrenia. The stress-vulnerability model postulates that an individual may have a predisposition to develop psychosis due to their genetic inheritance, birth complications, or early adversity in childhood that is associated with biological impacts on brain functioning. These propensities increase the likelihood of a psychotic episode occurring, but this is by no means a clearly predetermined pathway. It is only when environmental stressors interact with the underlying vulnerabilities that a psychotic episode may be triggered. Stressors can be of the obviously negative kind – poverty, bereavement, unemployment, a traumatic event, and so on – but it can also be an event that normally has positive connotations; for example, leaving home to go to university can sometimes be a trigger point for a psychotic illness in a young person who has an underlying genetic predisposition and a family history of psychosis. Although there are all sorts of methodological problems in conducting research in this area, the overall findings seem to be that individuals – particularly those with an enduring rather than episodic psychotic illness – are more likely than the general population to have had negative developmental experiences that include emotional, physical, or sexual abuse and neglect, as well as social stressors in adulthood; however, this adversity – so clearly important in the development of personality difficulties as we have shown in previous chapters – does not appear in itself to cause a psychotic illness without the presence of some underlying vulnerability.

Psychosis and the risk of violence

The debate has raged over the past few decades as to whether individuals with mental health problems, or those specifically with a psychotic illness, have a greater propensity to be violent than members of the general population. Box 8.2 sets out a summary of the key evidence from research that identifies the rates of violence towards others – and towards the self in terms of suicide – associated with individuals suffering from mental illness, but more specifically from a psychotic illness. The information is drawn from two sources: first, systematic reviews where the findings from multiple studies are collated in order to draw conclusions that are less biased by individual samples and methodological differences in the original research. Second, information has been drawn from the National Confidential Inquiry into Suicide and Safety in Mental Health (NCISH), managed by the University of Manchester and covering all suicides and – until recently – all homicides associated with individuals who have been under the care of mental health services during the year prior to the incident taking place.

As Box 8.2 shows, the risk of any violence in those who have a psychosis is around 10%, roughly five times greater than the risk in the general population; this is particularly marked for those with substance misuse problems, and indeed, it is substance misuse that accounts for most of the increased risk in those with psychosis. Although the public's perception may be that individuals with mental health problems are high risk for the most violent of offences – homicide – the actual annual figures are relatively small – around 50 individual cases per annum, accounting for approximately 10% of all homicides in the United Kingdom per annum. Every single one of these cases is a terrible tragedy and devastating for the families involved. Nevertheless, it is important to remember that the proportion of those with psychosis who go on to kill someone is tiny (3 in 1,000); however, such individuals are 15 times more likely to kill than a member of the general population. This is the same risk rate as individuals with substance misuse problems. There are numerous studies that have tried to identify what might be the features in individuals with

BOX 8.2

Evidence-based facts regarding psychosis and risk of violence

Violence

- Around 10% of individuals with psychosis are violent over their lifetime compared to 1.6% of the general population.
- The risk of violence is four times higher in those individuals with psychosis and substance misuse when compared to those with psychosis and no substance misuse.
- Violence, in those individuals with psychosis, is associated with:
    - A prior history of criminal convictions
    - Expressions of hostility towards others
    - Recent substance misuse
    - Non-compliance with medication

Homicide

- An average of around 50 homicides per year are perpetrated by those in contact with mental health services in the United Kingdom. This accounts for around 10% of all homicides per year.
- The risk of homicide perpetrated by an individual with psychosis is 0.3% (3 in 1,000). This is the same as the risk of homicide perpetrated by an individual with substance misuse problems only. The risk of homicide in the general population is 0.02%; therefore, the risk is 15 times higher in individuals with psychosis.

Suicide

- In 2017, 1,517 individuals under the care of mental health services took their lives. This accounted for 28% of suicides that year. Of these 1,517 patients,
    - 57% had a history of alcohol or drug misuse (866)
    - 13% had a history of psychosis (202)
- Six percent of individuals with psychosis will take their own life over their lifetime, therefore individuals with psychosis are 33 times more likely to take their own life than to take the life of someone else.

psychosis that are particularly associated with a heightened risk of violence: it is rare to find consistent evidence that particular aspects of the illness drive violence; rather, it seems that features with which we are already familiar from Chapter 7 on risk are emphasised: antisocial aspects of an individual's personality, and behaviours that could be considered to be secondary to personality features such as hostility, prior offending, substance misuse, and non-compliance. In this instance, non-compliance with the medication regime is particularly pertinent, as without medication, some individuals may well deteriorate in their mental health.

The picture in relation to suicide is rather different, insofar as around 1,500 individuals with mental health problems take their lives over the course of a year (the figures vary a little from year to year), around 200 of whom have a psychotic illness; again, substance misuse is particularly prevalent in this population.

What is the answer, therefore, to the question of the risk of violence linked to psychosis? The answer is mixed. The evidence is fairly robust in concluding that a psychotic illness or psychotic episode does indeed raise the risk of violence to others, but this increased risk is strongly linked to the individual with psychosis also misusing substances. Nevertheless, the vast majority of individuals with psychosis are not violent, and the risk of homicide is small; unfortunately, it is also true that the risk of homicide is much higher in this population than in the general population. Finally, and most significantly, the rate of suicide is tragically high in those with psychosis; that is, such individuals are 33 times more likely to take their own life rather than the life of another person.

How to understand the nature of the link: case histories

Facts and figures go some way to clarifying potential myths about the perceived dangerousness of psychotic individuals, but the issue only really takes on a meaning if we consider some case stories. Media reports tend to emphasise the bizarre and irrational in their accounts of psychotically driven violence, otherwise referring to 'motiveless' crimes, and sometimes hinting at the propensity of the individual perpetrator to malinger – exaggerating psychosis – in order to avoid the consequences of their actions. In reality, the nature of the link between psychosis and violence can be varied and complex. The following section is devoted to the description of four case vignettes, each narrative highlighting a different way in which a psychotic episode related to an act of violence. A simply explanatory model for this comprises the following:

- The symptoms of psychosis drive the violent offence.
- The violent offence occurs as mental health is deteriorating.
- The violent offence can be linked to negative symptoms.
- The violent offence has no relationship with the psychotic episode.

Peter's story: where the symptoms of psychosis drive the violent offence

Peter was aged 25 when he killed a sex worker; he was convicted of manslaughter (a lesser offence than murder in the eyes of the court) on the grounds of diminished responsibility and received a life sentence. The verdict was influenced by the expert testimony of psychiatrists who confirmed that Peter was psychotic at the time he killed the victim, and the killing was closely related to his mental state, such that he did not have full responsibility for his actions at the time.

Peter was not known to mental health services at the time of offence and had never been in contact with mental health previously. It was therefore necessary to put together an understanding of his decline into psychosis retrospectively, with the assistance of family members and Peter himself when his health improved. It seemed that Peter's upbringing had been fairly unremarkable, although a paternal grandfather had been known to have '*violent rages*' and '*crazy ideas*' which may, in hindsight, have been a sign of mental ill health. Peter was a rather quiet child, not very successful socially, but he was well-behaved, diligent at school, although not academically strong, and happy at home. The family was law-abiding and religious, his siblings were reasonably successful as adults.

Peter's decline in functioning seemed to start around the age of 20: he lost his job and struggled to find further employment, the family noticed that he took less care of his appearance and he was sometimes guarded in response to their questions about his well-being. He began to mention increasingly often that he needed to find a girlfriend, and could not understand why women seemed to shy away from him. Peter later revealed – although he was ashamed to admit it – that he started to frequent sex workers intermittently, and it seemed that he struggled to perform sexually at times as he suffered from impotence.

In the year or so prior to the offence, he changed the church he attended, choosing a Christian sect with a more charismatic approach to worship, and he approached his mother with concerns that someone had put '*the evil eye*' on him. Although Peter was British born, his mother had emigrated to the United Kingdom from West Africa, and he was familiar with her tales of the evil eye and spirit possession from her childhood days; although she believed in the power of the evil eye, she did not push her children to share her beliefs, and indeed they were rejected by all her children other than Peter. When he started to express these concerns, his mother, therefore, did not consider that he was in any way unstable.

Although Peter was guarded and did not fully share his thinking with others, by the time of the offence, he had become convinced that his impotence was related to the malicious intent of the victim who he believed was in liaison with the devil to put the evil eye on him. The victim was a sex worker who Peter had come to like as a rather kind and motherly figure who responded to his impotence in a sensitive way. Nevertheless, as we know from research studies, the person at risk is actually more likely to be someone in the psychotic individual's circle of friends and family, rather than a stranger. Peter became convinced of the victim's malicious intent, and in that context, felt that his well-being – if not his life as well – was at risk from her. He made an arrangement to meet her in the usual way, in her bedsit, but brought a knife with him, hidden on his person. He later denied that his intention was to kill her, although he was vague as to what exactly he intended to do, other than saying '*I wanted her to admit what she was doing, I think the knife was to threaten her, to frighten her into revealing her relationship with the devil*'. Nevertheless, it seems probable that he did not talk with her at the time as his retrospective account suggests, but immediately took out the knife and stabbed her once in the chest, piercing her heart; he ran out of the building and made his way to the local police station, immediately confessing to the police '*I've killed the devil*'.

In prison Peter responded well to medication for his psychotic illness, and gradually improved; it was for this reason that when he came to trial, he was considered well enough to manage a custodial sentence rather than a hospital order. The latter is a court sentence under the Mental Health Act (1983) in which an individual is ordered to spend time indefinitely in hospital until a Tribunal (and the Ministry of Justice, in some cases) deems them safe and well enough to release. In prison, Peter was thought to be eccentric, but not obviously unwell for much of the time, although some paranoid ideas came to the fore at times of particular stress (for example, when his mother died). He was maintained on medication, and managed to hold a simple prison job, cleaning on the wing. He took responsibility for his actions, in terms of the offence, and grudgingly accepted that his conclusions about the victim may have been somewhat misjudged (although he never fully relinquished his belief that spirit forces were in play).

Summarising the link between psychosis and violence in Peter's case, we can see that there is a direct relationship between his delusional belief – the victim maliciously imposing the evil eye on him in order to affect his sexual potency – and his violent act, the former driving the commission of the latter. Although personality difficulties are not obviously of any particular significance in understanding the offence in Peter's case, we can see that there are cultural influences to the content of his delusional beliefs. It is also difficult to discern whether his sexual difficulties were a precursor to the development of his delusional beliefs, or a consequence of increased anxiety associated with his deterioration in mental health, or perhaps entirely coincidental. It may surprise the reader to learn that this direct relationship between psychosis and violence is relatively rare; estimates vary but suggest that 10–40% of individuals with a psychotic illness and a violent offence fall into this category.

Quinn's story: the violent offence occurs as mental health is deteriorating

If Peter's story is relatively uncommon, then the example of Quinn will help to broaden our understanding of the way in which psychosis can link to violence. Quinn was aged 45 when he was convicted of indecent assault. His victim was his community psychiatric nurse (CPN) who – at the time of the offence – was interviewing him in the sitting room of the mental health hostel in which Quinn was living. There were concerns that had been raised by the hostel staff that Quinn was perhaps becoming mentally unwell again: staff had noticed that his self-care had been deteriorating, and he had become increasingly irritable – shouting at staff, unusually, when he made requests of them that were not immediately complied with; and they had noticed a smell of cannabis coming from his room, suggesting that he was perhaps smoking weed more than he had previously. The CPN usually visited every two to three weeks, but on both the previous visits, Quinn had slipped out of the hostel and could not be found and was therefore not seen. Nevertheless, he had attended a medical outpatient appointment with the psychiatrist a month before, who had found no evidence of psychotic symptoms such as auditory hallucinations or abnormal beliefs.

On the day of the offence, the CPN – who knew Quinn well – had planned the interview with the aim of trying to determine what was happening to Quinn's mental state; she had in mind the possibility that he was becoming psychotic, and there may be a need to bring him back into hospital for a more intensive assessment. However, the visit was difficult from the start, as Quinn was rather agitated, pacing up and down the room, mumbling to himself at times in a rather indistinct way; he then suddenly come up close to the nurse and asked her if she had a boyfriend. The nurse was taken aback, as this was most out of character for Quinn who was usually a quiet and rather polite individual who was respectful of patient-professional boundaries. She gently responded by reminding him that this was a private matter and not something she wanted to discuss with him; unfortunately, Quinn responded negatively to this feedback, and started to raise his voice at her. At the same time, and with no obvious trigger, he unzipped his trousers and exposed his penis; to her understandable alarm, he rushed towards her and grabbed her breast, repeatedly asking her *'have sex with me, have sex with me'*. The staff, having been waiting nearby in order to ensure the nurse's safety, heard the commotion and rushed into the room to help with the situation. Quinn retreated to the far side of the room, saying *'I just want sex, I didn't hurt her'*; and he allowed himself to be taken by a male key worker to a nearby room; by the time the police arrived, he was led away quite calmly.

Quinn's early life was difficult, as his father died when he was aged 8, and his mother struggled to cope with three children and the necessity of going out to work. She suffered from depression as a result, and was often emotionally unavailable to the children, although she managed to provide for them materially. Quinn left school at the age of 15, having previously truanted on a number of occasions; he was often found wandering around building sites – for which he acquired an early conviction for burglary – and was something of a loner, although liked well enough by his peers. He drifted through life to a large extent, having lost touch with his family, with intermittent work, and occasional intimate relationships, none of which were enduring. By the time he was 30, he had had a psychotic breakdown and was diagnosed with schizophrenia; excessive cannabis use was thought to have played a significant role in this breakdown. The following 15 years were characterised by admissions to hospital when he was psychotic, followed by periods of living in the community; initially he managed in independent accommodation, but he struggled to manage financially, and eventually lost his flat due to excessive rent arrears and difficulty complying with the support that he was offered. He had also received two separate prison sentences for fairly minor offences of robbery (snatching a woman's handbag), theft (stealing from shops), and a further burglary of a warehouse. Interestingly, he coped fairly well in prison, as his mental health was relatively stable on medication, he had no easy access to cannabis, and he enjoyed the regularity and predictability of the regime. The most recent – and rather lengthy – admission to hospital had occurred when he became psychotic, self-harmed, and then was found by the police on the cusp of throwing himself off one of the London bridges; he had then been placed in a 24-hour supported mental health hostel, where he had now resided for at least a year.

Piecing together the story of Quinn's deterioration prior to the offence of indecent assault, it became clear that the offence occurred within the context of a prodromal phase of decline into psychosis. The prodromal phase of a psychotic illness is the precursor phase to the development of frank psychotic symptoms such as those described in Box 8.1, the onset of which can be traced retrospectively back to the time at which an individual's functioning began to deteriorate. It is characterised by changes in mood, thinking, and behaviour – such as sleeplessness, agitation, low or elated mood, reduced personal grooming, suicidal thoughts, preoccupations, and so on – that suggest an individual is deteriorating. Psychological models tend to view this phase as a period of fragmentation or chaotic mental organisation that is frightening for the individual and which may lead to strenuous attempts to find meaning and personal control. Frank psychotic symptoms such as a delusional belief or hallucinations may provide a solution to such states of fragmentation, as although psychotic symptoms can sometimes be terrifying for an individual, they do at least bring meaning and sense to what otherwise feels like chaos. This simple theory then suggests that offences occurring within the prodromal phase – probably accounting for the majority of offending in those who are psychotic – represent a rather disorganised means by which individuals are trying to make sense of their deteriorating internal states of coherence.

In Quinn's case, two factors seemed to be at play in triggering this prodromal decline: his use of cannabis increased, probably including smoking stronger types of weed; and – as a search of his room later revealed – the hoarding of his medication to manage his mental illness. Most individuals in this situation would struggle to articulate this, even when restored to full health; for Quinn, it was his multidisciplinary team rather than he who made sense of his uncharacteristic assault on the nurse as an impulsive and rather incoherent attempt to act on this fragmentation of mind. That is, their understanding was that as Quinn deteriorated, he began to smoke more cannabis in an attempt to manage his increasing agitation; with increased cannabis use, his mental decline actually increased. Quinn began to think that his feelings of agitation could be soothed by sexual gratification – or at least we hypothesise that this is what he was thinking – and hence his disorganised sexual assault on the nurse.

The outcome for Quinn was relatively benign. The victim – his community nurse – was shaken but resilient, and remained at work. Quinn was taken to court and received a three-year community order, with a Mental Health Treatment Requirement. In essence, this meant that Quinn was under the supervision of the probation service for three years, and he had agreed to accept treatment as appropriate from his mental health team. Initially, he was resident in hospital as he had become frankly psychotic a few weeks after his arrest, with hostile voices commanding him to kill himself and he was thought to be at serious suicide risk; his medication was changed to depot (a slow release injection) rather than pills, given the previous hoarding behaviour. His mental health stabilised and he returned to the mental health hostel; he apologised to his nurse, but it was not felt appropriate that she resume care of him, and he was allocated a male community psychiatric nurse.

Rob's story: the violent offence can be linked to negative symptoms

Rob was aged 24 when he was convicted of grievous bodily harm, the victim being someone he had met in the park where a number of homeless individuals used to congregate and drink. Rob received a three-year custodial sentence for this offence, despite having a diagnosis of schizophrenia, as there was no indication that he was overtly psychotic at the time of the offence, and it was deemed reasonable that he receive a criminal justice sanction as he was willing to comply with his medication whilst in prison.

Rob's story was a rather poignant one: he had been a charming and mischievous child, perhaps a little quirky in his interests and his interactions with others, but always popular with his peers and his teachers. He seemed to be rather bright academically, and showed an interest in maths and sciences, and he had even talked of being a doctor or a research scientist at one point. He came from a settled and reasonably affluent family home, with working parents, family holidays by the sea, and plenty of affection. There was no indication of a problem until Rob moved from his local secondary school to a sixth form college slightly further away; he had chosen this move himself as the college specialised in science. Around the same time, his parents' marriage was in difficulty; his father had had an affair with someone at work, and there were increasing arguments at home. His mother was understandably and rather obviously upset, and the couple agreed to separate for a while. Rob took this news badly – as might any young person – but in his case, he seemed to struggle to keep this part of his life in perspective. He started missing days at college, and brooding in his bedroom, refusing to get out of bed; he was furious with his father and refused to maintain any contact with him, writing numerous angry emails to him that became increasingly threatening in tone. He then started to drink alcohol heavily, initially in the evenings, but increasingly during the day; this was a sensitive issue in the family as a maternal uncle had died of liver failure as a result of alcohol poisoning, and so Rob's parents became increasingly concerned about him.

Matters came to a crisis point, when Rob's behaviour became increasingly erratic, and his communications with his father frankly bizarre; one evening – heavily intoxicated – he tried to hang himself from the light shade in his room, but in the commotion, he was found by his mother before he was seriously hurt. Rob was taken to psychiatric hospital and admitted on an informal basis into a ward for observation. At that point he admitted to hearing voices, describing two unknown voices talking to each other in a derogatory way about his father, which Rob found intensely distressing. The mental health team concluded that he had suffered a psychotic episode and were moderately confident – quite understandably – that this may have been a one-off event following the stress of transitioning to college coinciding with the parental separation. With some counselling and medication, the voices seemed to abate, and Rob was discharged home.

However, his mother reported ongoing difficulties with Rob's social interactions and behaviour; she repeatedly said *'he's still not my Rob… my boy's not back with me'*: he was monosyllabic at home, his self-care was poor, he seemed uninterested in his former friends who all abandoned him one by one. Occasional flickers of interest in mechanics or science projects quickly came to nothing, as did talk of girlfriends and dates. Most distressing of all for the family was that Rob continued to drink heavily and they seemed to be unable to stop him; his parents restricted his allowance, but he stole off them; they hid their cash and credit cards, but he would verbally threaten them until they relented. Rob's sister – who was sitting her A-levels – started to suffer from anxiety as a result of the tension at home, and eventually Rob was asked to leave by his mother; he went to stay with his father for a while but this also became untenable, and a local authority studio flat was found for him.

At the time of the offence, Rob had simply abandoned his studio flat some months previously, with the vague intention of *'travelling'*, although he had no money and no plan. He became homeless, sometimes sleeping rough, sometimes in a homeless hostel. He continued to drink heavily and had been in trouble with the police for stealing money and/or alcohol on numerous occasions, as well as being convicted for affray six months earlier, after he had become embroiled in a fight with others over the ownership of a bottle of whiskey. The day of the offence was unremarkable; Rob entered the park with an empty can of lager in his hand with an intention of begging in order to buy a second can. He followed two or three people in the park, touching their sleeves and muttering *'money please'* in something of a monotone with a blank look on his face. People became understandably alarmed, although Rob did not appear to notice this and certainly did not react. He then approached another homeless man, and tried to take his can of drink off him; the other man resisted, and a brief scuffle ensued. Rob then walked away a few paces, turned and went back, and in quite a calm fashion, hit the man over the head with a bottle he had picked up, then stamping once on his head before walking away again. Later, Rob explained in a rather matter of fact tone *'I just needed to have a drink and he wouldn't help'*.

Box 8.1 outlines the negative symptoms that can be associated with an enduring psychotic illness. The reader can identify these 'absent' or 'deficit' symptoms in Rob's story; a narrative that is characterised by lack of some of the important features of personality that make us vibrantly individual. The tragedy – felt particularly keenly by his distressed parents – was the loss of personality that had ensued as a result of the illness. The reader may wonder why I stress the link between the violent offence and the negative symptoms as Rob was also a heavy drinker and it could be argued that he simply wanted money or drink that did not belong to him and became angry when thwarted. However, I would argue that there was no evidence for any strong negative emotion driving his offence. His behaviour in the park that day was symptomatic of his impoverished social skills, his lack of understanding of the emotional impact of his behaviour on others, the absence of any interpersonal strategy for managing conflict, and the curiously detached and slightly tangential response he ultimately demonstrated in response to resistance from the victim. This does not mean that Rob should not be held accountable to some extent for his actions and therefore be processed accordingly by the courts. However, discerning the disabling effects of an enduring psychotic illness, such as that suffered by Rob, is a fairly skilled task, and it would be unfair for his apparently cold and detached manner to be interpreted – in lay terms – as simply 'psychopathic' or 'remorseless'.

Stuart's story: the violent offence has no relationship with the psychotic episode

Stuart was aged 32 when he received an 18-year custodial sentence for three armed robberies; summarising his offending briefly, he had a long-standing dependency on crack cocaine, and was habitually in and out of prison for acquisitive offences that he committed in order to fund his use of drugs. The index offences were committed on a series of off licences, Stuart using a shotgun to threaten the shop assistants.

Stuart's early life was, as might now be expected by the reader, a problematic one: his father was also a habitual criminal, and his mother struggled to control the children that she was bringing up on her own during the long periods when her husband was absent. The boys – Stuart was one of three – all had reputations in the neighbourhood and at school as wild and rough boys with a dangerous father, and a tendency to cause trouble wherever they went. In adolescence, each boy followed the older into gangs where they were introduced to a range of illegal substances and criminal behaviour. It was not so much that Stuart had experienced adversity or trauma as his world view was so distorted from a very early age; his only role models were his father – surrounded by criminal mystique – and his delinquent peers. By his 20s, Stuart was a domineering and rather ruthless criminal who had lost control of his growing drug use, although he was not yet ready to admit as such.

Stuart embarked on his very long prison sentence without any sign that his mental state was fragile. He behaved as everyone expected him to – disobeying orders, subverting the authority of prison officers, seeking out other antisocial peers, and domineering the more vulnerable prisoners – and he was generally thought of as a rather unlikeable character. It was only two years into his sentence that Stuart's behaviour began to change; the changes were initially subtle, and it was probably almost a year before concerns really escalated. Initially Stuart appeared to become rather low in mood and preoccupied – in a way that seemed entirely reasonable if out of character – with the length of his sentence; he was occasionally found crying in his cell. Then his behaviour became increasingly erratic: he started to tape newspaper over his windows and he was repeatedly reprimanded for doing the same over his cell door hatch. He also went through periods of refusing to eat prison food, subsisting entirely on packets of biscuits and noodles that he bought for himself; there were occasional notes in the prison record that he had referred to the food being contaminated, and he started to show a suspicious attitude towards healthcare staff who came to assess his mental state. Eventually, there was an occasion when the staff insisted on a cell search and found that he had written 'help' on the wall by his bed in what appeared to be blood. He was transferred – completely against his will – to the inpatient unit in the prison. Staff held polarised views: some believed that he was malingering in order to obtain privileges or even a transfer to hospital, others felt that he was suffering from a drug-induced psychosis, possibly induced by Spice[1] use. Ultimately, the view that he was psychotic prevailed, but as Stuart refused to take any medication to manage his psychotic state – and medication cannot be enforced in prison – it was agreed that he should be transferred to a secure hospital for treatment.

Stuart was transferred to hospital under a section of the 1983 Mental Health Act. He eventually seemed to settle in hospital, and although medication had to be enforced initially, he was subsequently compliant. The nurses thought of him as a rather anxious and frightened individual who kept himself to himself; there was no sign of the domineering and bullying Stuart they had heard about from prison staff. He participated in the ward programme of therapeutic activities and was gradually given a little more freedom, which he managed without incident; eventually, he was allowed to have a 30-minute walk in the hospital grounds with a nurse as escort. It was on the third day of his walk in the grounds that Stuart suddenly ran off from the nurse and dashed out of the hospital. Piecing events together much later on, it seemed that he was able to hitch a ride with a van driver and managed to disappear into an urban underworld of *'invisible people'* (as he put it). Stuart was eventually found by the police a month later, sleeping rough in an underpass; he was patently terrified when he saw them and struggled when they arrested him shouting *'save me'*, clearly in fear of his life. He was returned to high-secure prison – as a potential escape risk – and immediately transferred to the hospital wing of the prison as he was very obviously psychotic, with persecutory beliefs that a complex web of people – including the hospital staff – were intending to kill him. Later, Stuart was able to describe his state of mind at the time of his hospital transfer and subsequent escape from care with great clarity. He said that he realised there was a plot to kill him, and that he was very unsafe in the hospital, the caring nature of the staff being a particularly dangerous ploy to lull him into a false sense of security. Terrified, he was therefore hyper-alert to potential risk and realised he needed to pretend that he was well in order to instigate a return to prison where he felt he would be better able to protect himself. Although this view did not entirely accord with his decision to abscond from the hospital, it seemed to make sense to him at the time; he carefully planned the escape, hoarding money and identifying where he might best find a lift into the town. He said he chose to live with a varying group of eccentric and disturbed homeless men in the rabbit warren of railway arches in the urban centre, existing on end-of-the-day scraps of food from soup kitchens and stolen bottles of cheap alcohol.

Interestingly, as Stuart gradually improved in the prison healthcare wing – taking his medication regularly as he had been so frightened by his state of mind when psychotic – his former persona started to reappear. The staff began to comment that they 'preferred Stuart ill' as he began to extort money and favours from other healthcare patients, and to treat the nursing staff with some disdain, distancing himself from the patient role. He returned to the main wing and remained in mainstream location for the following ten or so years, progressing to conditions of lower security, and eventually applying to the Parole Board for release. He had come off medication around five years earlier and there had been no sign of any relapse.

The example of Stuart clearly shows how someone who had been habitually violent when mentally well shifted from being rather unlikeable and antisocial to a fragile and needy individual beset with terrifying psychotic experiences when unwell. His psychotic state was absolutely not characterised by violence, and his dramatic escape and later response to being rearrested was driven by terror and a fear for his life. It will probably never be entirely clear what triggered Stuart's rather drawn-out psychotic episode: it may have been an unusually extreme depressive episode that tipped him into psychosis, or the result of the highly unpredictable effects of Spice or a similar new psychoactive substance (referred to as NPS). My own view is that it was probably a combination of the two: I think it is likely that Stuart began to face up to the reality of his extremely long prison sentence, and he became depressed; when combined with the dangerously unpredictable NPS – something he probably smoked more of as his mood dropped with the result that his psychotic experiences were exacerbated – a vicious circle of interactions occurred that triggered an enduring psychotic state.

Summary

What lessons does this chapter provide? Although mental illness is a broad subject, we have focused here on one of the most serious aspects of the experience – psychosis and its relationship to the risk of violence. I imagine that the reader is both reassured and alarmed by the facts presented here, as well as having perhaps a more emotional response to the four narratives provided. To remind the reader, it is certainly the case that there is a heightened risk of violence – including homicide – associated with individuals who are suffering from psychosis, but this risk is as much to do with the antisocial features of the individuals' behaviour and their substance misuse, as the mental state itself. Much more likely – and something that is less in the public's vision – is the risk of suicide in such individuals. These facts feed into something that goes beyond the scope of this chapter, which is the unsettling and established link between mental illness and a severely reduced life expectancy in the individual.

I hope that the four case narratives – albeit linked as they are in various ways to acts of serious violence – show a more poignant and meaningful side to the struggles of individuals who are psychotic and violent. These narratives also touch on the challenges with which mental health services can be faced, and hint at the devastation that follows terrible events; victims and their loved ones are foremost in our minds, but there is no doubt that the lives of the perpetrators are also characterised by struggle and their loved ones also suffer.

Note

1. Spice is a new psychoactive substance that is sometimes referred to as 'synthetic marijuana', comprising a mix of herbs and laboratory-made chemicals.

Further reading

The best source of information on suicide and homicide associated with mental illness is the National Confidential Inquiry into Suicide and Safety in Mental Health, including their annual reports and publications linked to their research studies:

https://sites.manchester.ac.uk/ncish/

Epidemiology studies are those that take large populations samples to explore prevalence rates of particular issues; systematic reviews of smaller studies are also important. There are a range of studies, but a starting point would be the following:

Fazel, S., Gulati, G., Linsell, L., Geddes, J.R., & Grann, M. (2009). Schizophrenia and violence: systematic review and meta-analysis. *PLoS Medicine*, 6, 100–120. http://dx.doi.org/10.1371/journal.pmed.1000120

Witt, K., van Dorn, R., and Fazel, S. (2013). Risk factors for violence in psychosis: systematic review and meta-regression analysis of 110 studies. *PLoS One*, 8, https://doi.org/10.1371/journal.pone.0055942

Hundred Families is an organisation that campaigns, provides information, and raises awareness from the perspective of family and loved ones who are bereaved by an individual with mental health problems. www.hundredfamilies.org

Tom, Vic, and William's story 9

Fantasy, planning, and 'seemingly irrelevant decisions'

Tom's story

I would encourage the reader to go through the following dialogue with an open mind, noticing your reactions as the story develops, and then perhaps to reread it in light of the subsequent discussion on 'seemingly irrelevant decisions'.

TOM I've told people the story so many times; yes, I had sex with her, yes, I now realise that she wasn't fully willing and that's my fault, I admit it. But it was just one of those things, it happened, I didn't go out that night looking for a woman to rape, I'm not that sort of guy. I've been called a 'predatory rapist', what does that mean? … I don't think about women that way, I don't struggle to find women, I'm – or I was – just a good time sort of bloke, out with my mates that night. I thought I was going to get laid, we had sex, she cried, I left her flat; it's like the whole sorry tale took about 15 minutes from start to finish.

PSYCHOLOGIST I appreciate the fact that when you went out that evening, rape was not on your mind; our previous conversation helped me to understand that. But if I were to ask you at exactly what moment that evening did you know that you were going to rape the victim, what would you say?

TOM That's my point, it was never in my mind, I never said to myself 'ah, now I'm going to rape you', it just wasn't like that. I suppose I would say that when she started to cry, I knew something was wrong, I had an uneasy feeling in my gut, and I made sure I left pretty quick after that.

PSYCHOLOGIST So I think what we need to work out is how, at one moment you're going out for a normal fun evening with mates, and only a few hours later, you're in a position where you're going to get a ten-year prison sentence. ... Let's try and make sense of it, let's start with you going out that evening. What was on your mind?

TOM It was a normal Saturday, I had a few drinks in my local, a couple of lines (of cocaine) – I'm not apologising for that, we all partied at the weekend in those days. I met some friends at the club, and we were just having a good time, a bit of dancing and all that.

PSYCHOLOGIST Were you a mixed group of male and female friends?

TOM No, just my male mates, none of us were seriously attached, we were just looking for a good time.

PSYCHOLOGIST When you say not attached, and 'a good time', I'm assuming that you were thinking you might get lucky that night, perhaps pick up a woman and sleep with her? Or am I being unfair?

TOM Not unfair, no. But we weren't looking to rape anyone if that's what you're thinking. Yeah, we might get lucky, I generally had no trouble finding a girl who wanted a good time too.

PSYCHOLOGIST So tell me a bit about what happened. ...

TOM So we were having fun, dancing and all that, and I saw the girl, she smiled at me, and I bought her a drink, and we danced some more. She was pretty lively, she asked me about pills so I assumed she was up for it, and ...

PSYCHOLOGIST Sorry to interrupt, but can I pause you there, and just ask you a couple of things? It sounds like you feel the girl made the first move in some way, and that her question about pills meant what exactly?

TOM So she was on her own, the smile was a signal definitely, no doubt. She was kind of ok but plump and on her own, no way was she going to get picked up without giving out a bit of encouragement.

PSYCHOLOGIST Would it be fair to say that you thought this was going to be an easy pick up?

TOM Yes, I suppose so, although you make it sound nasty. She was her own person, a bit high but in control, maybe an easy pull, that's what I thought at the time.

PSYCHOLOGIST So what happened?

TOM Nothing, I went to get her another drink, and she disappeared, left.

PSYCHOLOGIST Hmmm, what went through your mind at that point?

TOM I was pissed off.

PSYCHOLOGIST You'd bought her two drinks, and she owed you?

TOM Well not exactly. ... Well yes I suppose so, kind of. ... I was frustrated, my mates were laughing at me...

PSYCHOLOGIST Actually laughing, or you thought they might laugh?

TOM The second one, but she had made me look stupid, but I thought 'silly cow' and dismissed her.

PSYCHOLOGIST And then what happened next?

TOM So, I decided to cut my losses, my cousin had said to go over to his place, and there was nothing happening at the club. So I left… I needed to buy cigarettes before heading over to my cousin's. So I took a detour and there she was, a bit ahead of me, walking.

PSYCHOLOGIST Can I just stop you and ask about the 'detour' you mentioned. Were you looking for her at that point?

TOM Not intentionally, but I suppose it was in the back of my mind that maybe I would see her. …

PSYCHOLOGIST And when you saw her?

TOM I swear that the only thought in my head at that moment was that I would invite her to my cousin's house … and that's all I did, I caught up with her and we got chatting again.

PSYCHOLOGIST Was she pleased to see you?

TOM She didn't try to get away from me if that's what you mean. But she was pretty cool, I would say, at that point, and she said she was tired and wanted to go home. I didn't think that was right really, it was 4a.m., she was pissed or high or something, and I wasn't going to leave her alone, so I said I'd walk her to her flat.

PSYCHOLOGIST I'm sure you know what I'm going to ask you now.

TOM There was no way I thought 'hey I know, I'll rape her'.

PSYCHOLOGIST No, but perhaps you thought she might be willing to have sex with you?

TOM Ok, so maybe I thought I was in with a chance, why otherwise would she let me walk with her, I knew she probably liked me, letting me buy her drinks, walk her home, and all that.

PSYCHOLOGIST And when you got to the flat?

TOM She made some lame excuse about being tired, and tried to shut her front door.

PSYCHOLOGIST And we know that at that point, you stuck your foot in the door, and then pushed it back open and walked in. So I've got a sense of what might have been in your mind just then, but I don't want to put words in your mouth, you tell me what you think was going on for you at that exact moment.

TOM I was surprised and annoyed … no, I was angry, I thought 'you teasing c***', no you don't, not now, not after stringing me along all evening.

PSYCHOLOGIST So that was the moment that you knew you were going to rape her.

This chapter explores the moments – whether brief or prolonged – that form a bridge between the developing context for or triggers to an offence with the act of violence itself. Fantasy, planning, and 'seemingly irrelevant decisions' (SIDs) lie somewhere on a continuum between unconscious and conscious decision-making that creates opportunities to offend. They are important aspects of the narrative for many individuals who have committed acts of serious violence, as they enable us to understand the meaning of the violent act in a much more holistic way than simply making assumptions about motivation based on common sense. Tom's story – a highly condensed example of a dialogue between him and a psychologist – exemplifies the role of SIDs in understanding offending behaviour. If we accept that Tom may not have fulfilled the role of 'predatory rapist' as had been said of him, then we need to be curious about his thinking on that night of the rape. Why, you may feel, does this matter; and why, you may think even more strongly, can we not simply conclude that Tom's attitudes towards women are derogatory and unacceptable and need to be changed? It is certainly true that for many individuals, understanding the details of thoughts and feelings leading up to an offence may not be that important in managing risk going forwards. We have already seen that those individuals who maintain denial of their offence do not pose a higher risk than those who can articulate their offence details. We also know that trying to change generally distorted or unhelpful attitudes by verbal challenge is largely unsuccessful, leads to hostile stand-offs between practitioner and offender; and has a limited impact on any future risk.

We all employ SIDs in particular contexts: consider, for example, the alcoholic who realises that he needs cigarettes after the closing time of the local shop, necessitating a trip to the cigarette machine in the local pub; alternatively, consider the person on a diet who – after a session at the gym – decides to take the long route home which happens to pass the bakery. In both examples, individuals may deny any intent to 'lapse' and their thinking is outside conscious awareness, but nevertheless we can recognise the behaviours as facilitating a 'lapse' – and in the latter example, we might hypothesise that in the back of the person's mind, is a belief that they are 'owed a treat' for having been virtuous in the gym. Identifying and challenging these SIDs may form an important component of any relapse prevention approach.

In Tom's case, I would suggest that he probably does need to understand how he went from *'good time guy'* to *'rapist'* in a few hours; his initial appraisal that the offence *'just happened'* is a common one; it is not true, but at the same time, Tom may be speaking from the heart. What the condensed dialogue suggests – although in reality, requiring several sessions to fully disentangle – is that Tom made a large number of SIDs on the evening of the offence that enabled him to move from feckless flirt to determined rapist, without him ever consciously planning to rape a woman until the moment he stuck his foot in the door that the victim was trying to shut. For example, he expected to have sex, he targeted a woman he considered to be '*easy*', he took her departure as a personal humiliation and disrespectful given that she '*owed him*'; he altered his route to his cousin's house for spurious reasons, and he reinterpreted the victim's '*cool*' attitude and acquiescence as consent to sex rather than an indication of unease or fear, ultimately leading to his sense of entitlement when he pushed into her flat and raped her. Summarised in one sentence, we might conclude that although Tom's *plan* was to have sex that night, his *SIDs* led him to rape the victim.

The role of deviant sexual interests and pornography in planning sexual offending

In Chapter 4, we considered the difference between instrumental and reactive aggression, recognising that for some individuals, aggression could be premeditated and intentional in order to achieve a goal; for others, aggression might be triggered by a perceived threat suggesting an impulsive response to a negative feeling. With those who commit sexual offences, we are more likely to assume that the primary aim of the act is sexual and that the precursor may well include a relevant sexual fantasy – whether it comprises sexual arousal to an imagined or real child, or sexual arousal to the act of aggressive sex with an unwilling adult. However, evidence suggests that this deviancy or addiction model has rather limited value; not only do a significant number of individuals – such as Tom – object to these assumptions, but the variable reoffending and reconviction rate for those with sexual offences suggests that a range of motivations are at play. If the range of sexual reconviction rates is 3–60% over 10–20 years at risk in the community,[1] then even though we may have doubts about the truth of these figures, we can conclude that some men are more driven than others to repeat their offending, despite the drastic consequences if caught. This leads us to speculate that the role of fantasy in offending is focused on risk – the question as to whether thinking about sexual behaviour increases the likelihood of that sexual behaviour being enacted – and is best examined in the first instance by understanding the debate on the role of pornography in offending behaviour.[2] That is, to what extent does engaging in sexual fantasies by the viewing of pornography increase the sexual interest in and planning of sexual offences?

Box 9.1 outlines the relevant definitions for pornography and fantasy, although a quick perusal of internet search engines suggests that definitions can be rather varied; a few options are provided, each with slightly different

BOX 9.1

Definitions of pornography and fantasy

Pornography is...

- The portrayal of sexual subject matter for the exclusive purpose of sexual arousal
- The depiction of erotic behaviour intended to cause sexual excitement

Fantasy is....

- The activity of imagining impossible or improbable things
- To imagine the occurrence of something
- To create something from one's imagination that is not based on reality

An ***extreme pornographic image*** is of such a nature that:

1. It must reasonably be assumed to have been produced solely or principally for the purpose of sexual arousal, and is
2. Grossly offensive, and
3. Portrays in an explicit and realistic way acts which involve rape (or bestiality or necrophilia – sex with dead bodies etc.)

Child sexual abuse images (formerly known as child pornography) is....

- A form of child exploitation involving any depiction of sexually explicit conduct involving a minor (aged less than 18) (USA)
- An indecent photograph of someone under the age of 18, in which indecency can be classified as such if the child is naked and the photograph emphasises their genitals, for example, not just that the photograph depicts sexual activity (UK)

use of language. Although every effort is made to be objective in the courts in relation to extreme pornography and child sexual abuse images, it is immediately apparent that there is room for personal and cultural differences in interpretation of these concepts. In particular, there is room for dispute regarding the boundary between erotic art and pornography (although the stated difference is whether the primary aim is artistic, or for the purposes of sexual arousal) and differences between the intention of the producer versus the interest of the viewer. As a rather niche example, a man with a shoe fetish may find a shoe catalogue intensely sexually arousing even though the intent of the catalogue producers was simply to induce a desire to purchase shoes.

The debate about pornography and its impact on male behaviour in particular has raged for decades. More recently, with the universal availability of the internet, the debate has intensified as an explosion in availability and viewing of online pornography has become apparent. The range of methodologies and findings make summarising the research rather complex. However, the simplified conclusion is that there is no real evidence that pornography use – including extreme pornography use – increases the likelihood of a sexual crime; there is some evidence that frequent pornography use is associated with more negative attitudes towards women and endorsement of derogatory or distorted beliefs about women and sex (although this is an association rather than a clear causal relationship). What this provides is yet further evidence that there is something of a disconnect between attitudes and behaviour, at least for the average person.

It is important to add that there are particular subgroups of individuals who have been found to be more vulnerable to the influences of pornography than others. First, those individuals who have already acquired a conviction for a sexual offence against a child have been found to pose a higher risk of sexual reconviction if they use pornography – in this case, the downloading and viewing of child sex abuse images. This makes intuitive sense: if someone has a sexual interest in children, and indulges in sexual fantasies about children – fuelled by viewing pornography – they may be more likely to seek out a child with whom to enact their fantasy. Second, there are understandable concerns about the influence of pornography on young people who currently have unprecedented access to a range of sexual imagery on the internet. Again research in this area does not indicate that teenagers are increasingly engaging in any of the specialist areas – even if legal –of sexual interest that they may be viewing. Interestingly, the research shows that high frequency use of pornography by teenagers is associated with unrealistic expectations about partner attractiveness, reduced sexual satisfaction in relationships, and difficulty sustaining such relationships. As yet, there is no indication of a raised risk of aggressive sexual behaviour.

If the research suggests a relatively weak influence of pornography – that is, the supply of sexual fantasy material – on behaviour, what do we make of the explosion of convictions for the downloading of child abuse images – formerly referred to as child pornography. Surely, it would be reasonable to expect those who download and view such images to have a strong sexual interest in children and to be at risk for acting on such sexual interests, in terms of seeking out and sexually assaulting children? The recorded crime figures would suggest that we are suffering from an epidemic of paedophilia if that is the case: for example, in relation to recorded crime in England and Wales from April 2018 to March 2019, there were 17,521 obscene publication offences against children recorded (equating to around 400–450 arrests in the United Kingdom each month), and during that same year, the UK Child Abuse Image Database (CAID) added a further 2,000,000 images to the database. Although these crime figures do not represent individual people (as one person may be convicted of several offences), it does nevertheless suggest that there are thousands of people – almost all men – for whom we should expect the outcome to be poor in terms of sexual reconviction. This has been assiduously studied in the past ten years, and the outcomes are fairly consistent. Of those convicted of child sexual abuse image offences, around 15% have previous convictions for a contact sexual offence – such as indecent assault – and therefore represent child sexual abusers who have reoffended. However, around 80% or so of the internet offenders have no prior sexual convictions; when followed up for at least four years in the community, the findings of meta-analyses suggest that around 5% reoffend in exactly the same way – downloading child abuse images – and around 2% escalate their behaviour to a further sexual offence that involves physical contact with a victim. These are *not* the findings we would expect to see if our assumptions about deviant sexual interests and subsequent behaviour were correct; we would expect to find a much higher rate of escalation to a contact sex offence with a child. One suggestion is that these individuals represent 'closet paedophiles' – individuals who would like to have sexual relations with a child but do not do so for a variety of reasons. Certainly, this fits for a minority; however, once one starts to hear the individual narratives that describe the pathway to offending, we begin to realise that for many, they have pursued a pathway in which the offence – viewing illegal images – has a function that is more complex than sexual gratification alone. That is, the fantasy enables the individual to manage an underlying problematic emotional state, it provides temporary relief or offers a temporary soothing effect, but fails to resolve the emotional difficulty and therefore propels the individual into a rather compulsive sequence of repetitive viewing behaviours. Some of the most commonly described narratives in relation to child sexual abuse imagery are as follows:

- Having habituated in adolescence and early adulthood to the use of pornography as a substitute for intimacy, the individual constantly seeks more exciting and subsequently more 'forbidden' sexual imagery in order to maintain the addictive 'hit'.
- In the context of a life crisis – unemployment, relationship breakdown, serious health scare – the individual seeks solace from a fantasy world that momentarily acts as 'antidepressant' providing a soothing and comforting effect.

- The individual is troubled by his own personal trauma – often child sexual abuse – and is drawn to seek answers by exploring child sexual abuse imagery, repeating and reversing scenarios of abuse (see Chapter 5 for more explanation of these ideas).

Understanding the role of fantasy in regulating self-esteem

In the above section, we came to understand that fantasy may have meaning beyond an imagined rehearsal of the act as a precursor to action. As Box 9.2 outlines, fantasy should not be thought of restrictively as only sexual; this is a mistake commonly made with individuals with sexual convictions, where it is assumed that the only relevant fantasies are sexual in nature. The examples drawn from the narratives of individuals who download illegal child abuse images suggest that meaning may relate to how the individual feels about themselves and/or how the individual processes negative emotional states. In this section, we explore further the way in which fantasy provides clues as to the meaning of the violent offence. To understand this, we need to start by exploring the relationship between the role of fantasy and self-esteem for all of us (see Box 9.2). Many of us spend hours engaged in fantasy each day, but we refer to it as daydreaming, imagination, visualisation, creative thought, inventiveness, and so on. Let us consider a very simple scenario – job interviews. Clearly, many of us would think about a forthcoming interview and anticipate the questions that might be asked; we would *rehearse* the interview in our minds in advance. However, for some of us, we might feel quite despondent about our current low-paid and low-status job, and imagine what it would be like to have a high-powered important job; we might spend hours imagining ourselves as prime minister, or as a heroic heart surgeon, for example. These are fantasies – what I refer to as superhero fantasies – in which our imagination engages in wish-fulfilling or escapist fantasies that *boost our self-esteem*, even though they may be entirely unrealistic. However, consider the job interview that went badly, the aggressive questioning that left us floundering and humiliated, and the subsequent rejection. For many of us, we need to engage in a series of fantasies – or imaginings – that enable us to *restore our self-esteem*; these often involve scenarios that turn the tables, imagining our witty and incisive responses to the aggressive questions, which now leave the interviewer humiliated.

If the example of job interviews feels remote, then consider our use of fantasy in relation to intimate relationships: we have probably all rehearsed what we might say to persuade someone to go on a date; we have adored someone from afar – albeit they were unattainable, perhaps even a

BOX 9.2

The role of fantasy in regulating self-esteem

FANTASY AS A REHEARSAL

The function of fantasy is to rehearse and plan a scenario that is intended to be enacted. With a sexual offence, the fantasy is of the offence to be committed, and it fuels the subsequent assault.

FANTASY AS A BOOST TO SELF-ESTEEM

The function of fantasy is to raise self-esteem from a lower level, by means of escapist or wish-fulfilment scenarios in which the individual is imagined as powerful and admired. With a sexual offence, the fantasy is seductive or 'romantic' in content, the subjective experience of the perpetrator as feeling inadequate in relationship terms, and despite the objective experience of the assault as unwanted and frightening by the victim.

FANTASY AS RESTORING SELF-ESTEEM

The function of fantasy is to repair or restore a sense of self-esteem back to its former level, after experiences that have been experienced as an attack on one's self-esteem. With a sexual offence, the fantasy is primarily vengeful, and the driving emotion in the offence is angry, the sexual element demonstrating a need to humiliate or terrorise the victim.

celebrity – and imagined a romantic wish-fulfilment scenario with them; and we might have responded to a humiliating rejection from a partner with vengeful fantasies that aimed to 'teach them a lesson', perhaps involving an infidelity or a put down.

Understanding the differential function of our imagination (or fantasy life) in regulating our self-esteem then leads us to consider how we might apply this understanding to violent offending; Box 9.2 outlines how, from a theoretical point of view, we can understand fantasy in relation to violent offences, but it feels very abstract without examples. The following case vignettes of two men convicted of rape offences against adult women provide a glimpse into the internal world of the rapist.

Vic's story

Vic was 35 years old and serving an eight-year prison sentence for attempted rape and assault (occasioning actual bodily harm – ABH) on a woman who he did not know but had followed one evening as she walked home from the shops late at night, and then attacked on her doorstep. He had a previous conviction for indecent exposure going back to when he was aged 22, an incident that he had always previously explained away as having been caught urinating in a park when he was drunk one night. He was a rather quiet and withdrawn character, very inarticulate when it came to describing his feelings, although intellectually quite able. However, when he referred himself to a prison therapeutic community – motivated to understand his offence and to make something of his life when released – his offence narrative began to develop, and the central role of fantasy in his offence became clearer.

Vic's childhood had not been an unhappy experience characterised by abuse, as so many of his peers in the therapeutic community had described; yet he had been disturbed by his experiences in the family home and had been a 'poor fit' with his parents in terms of personality. His parents were an exuberant and – for the times in which they lived – rather exotic couple, wrapped up in an intense emotional and sexual relationship with each other. Vic described his mother as *'stunningly beautiful ... she was so alluring, you just wanted to touch her, be with her or next to her. It was like being bathed in a warm glow'*. Although he used uniquely positive words to describe her – and was resistant to any question of criticism – it also became clear that she could not resist using her seductive powers on her son, and she would flirt with him in a way that made him feel uncomfortable, particularly during his adolescence when she was frank and explicit in teasing him when he had an erection; she used to refer to his masturbatory fantasies under the guise of sexual openness, but in reality, with a slightly taunting edge to her questioning that was insensitive to his embarrassment. His father was a more austere character, a handsome ex-soldier, who worked long hours in the financial sector, and devoted himself to his wife with whom he was extremely preoccupied. This preoccupation did not take the form of jealousy, as can often be the case, but was characterised by constant physical touching and overt emotional intensity that – as Vic later acknowledged – *'left no place for me in that family'*. It took Vic many months of therapy to be able to articulate his strenuous childhood attempts to be noticed and accepted by his father, all of which were met by indifference or – occasionally – overt rejection. Despite this lack of attention and affection directed towards Vic, his parents prided themselves on their natural approach to sex, and so there was a home environment characterised by sexually frank conversation, available pornography, nudity, and some suggestion of sexual role play and 'swinging'.[3] With puberty, Vic learnt to turn to sex and sexual fantasy as a source of gratification, and this quickly became a substitute for affectionate bonds and a feeling of belonging; he had always struggled to forge relationships with peers – although he was increasingly sought out by girls at school as a sort of platonic confidant, a 'good listener' with whom they discussed their dating problems. Vic increasingly retreated into his internal world, a world in which he was a strong and powerful seducer of women.

Vic struggled to make any significant impression on the world in his young adulthood; he made his way in life – studying and then working – and had a few fairly insipid and unsuccessful attempts at forging sexual relationships with women. However, the more insignificant he felt himself to be '*in the real world*', the greater the draw of his internal world. It was in this context – and indeed, he was drunk that night – that he '*found myself in the park, exposing my penis to this woman who was walking past*'. At that time, Vic persuaded himself that perhaps he was urinating, or it had been an unfortunate accident with his flies open at the wrong moment. Later in prison, he was gradually able to work out that he had had some sort of '*seduction fantasy ... I think I thought she was going to see my penis, see me wanking, and sort of. ... I'm embarrassed to say it now ... sort of be impressed. You know, laugh maybe, get turned on ... go home and fantasise about me and how much she wanted me.... [I]t sounds crazy now, but that's what I think I was thinking*'. The court sanction was minor – a conditional discharge – and Vic and his family filed away the incident in their minds as an embarrassing mistake. However, over the next few years, Vic's fantasy life developed as his external life remained static; he increasingly became focused on fantasies that enabled him to overcome the woman's initial resistance; he rarely watched pornography, but if he did, he was always watching the woman's facial expression, looking for signs that she desired the man, that she was acquiescent – despite her protestations. In the elaborate fantasies that he created himself and that took up much of his barren leisure time, he was always seeking the perfect romantic union with a woman, and this seemed more achievable if he had to overcome the woman's resistance and her denial of his seductive power in the initial struggle.

Vic spent a good deal of time in therapy in prison trying to work out what tipped him from being a fantasist into becoming a perpetrator. He looked back on the dismal quality of his life at that time, and wondered to what extent he was depressed or felt that he could not carry on in that way indefinitely; however, he was so wrapped up in his fantasies at the time that even in retrospect he was not able to identify an awareness of any negative emotional state. He also considered the role that his new female neighbour may have played – quite inadvertently – as her confident and mildly flirtatious manner reminded him slightly of his mother. Drink also contributed – although he was never a heavy drinker – as it took the '*edge off my inhibitions*' – and he was mildly intoxicated on the night of the offence. On the first night, Vic spotted the victim as she walked home from the high street, and he followed her; he openly admitted that following her gave him '*quite a buzz*', and he began to think about the possibility of enacting his fantasies with her. The second night, he waited around for her but was disappointed not to see her; he described something of a reality check that evening, and vowed that he would stop. Several days passed but by this time he was utterly preoccupied with the possibility of seeking out the victim, fully convinced that she would become the love of his life. He went out again to wait for her, spotted her, and followed her home. At some point he saw her smile, and '*knew*' that this was the signal, and that he simply needed to overcome her initial resistance; at the door step he grabbed her and forced her against her front door, fully intending to '*seduce her*' without her consent. He then described his amazement and shock when she started to scream and cry, clearly in intense distress and fear; initially he covered her mouth with his hand and in doing so, banged her head hard against the wall, but then he described it '*as though I was waking up from a dream… I was angry with her. What was she doing? … and then I started to think what am I doing? I felt completely confused, anxious, and I ran off*'.

Incredible as it may seem, Vic's offence was fuelled by intensely romantic notions of seduction and perfect union that would have appeared as offensively unrealistic to the victim had she known what was in his mind at the time he attacked her. Although ultimately Vic's fantasies were not enough to satisfy him, they had served an important function for many years, providing a vivid internal world that raised his self-esteem and created a '*super seducer*' in contrast to the sense of inadequacy and bleakness of his external world. The therapeutic regime at the prison, with the emphasis on group therapy with his male peers, forced Vic to focus on his emotional understanding of himself – rather than rely on sexual fantasies to regulate his self-image – and helped him to develop a stronger sense of himself in relation to his peers. Key elements to managing his risk, as he eventually progressed towards the community, included managing his alcohol use, but largely targeted the need for him to develop a stronger commitment to and improved skills in living in the 'real world' – friendships, work, leisure interests, and so on – and relinquishing his comforting 'fantasy world'.

For William, whose narrative we now consider, the role of fantasy was quite different; for him, fantasy was about vengeance; a terror of abandonment that led him to imagine scenarios in which he held total control and dominance over the victim in ways that functioned to restore his self-esteem.

William's story

William was aged 40 when he received a discretionary life sentence with a tariff[4] of 12 years for three rape convictions, each of which was committed during the course of a burglary and all of which took place over a two-year period before he was caught. As with Vic, William had also sought help from a prison therapeutic community, although it took him eight years to decide to take this step, and a further two years before he was able to open up with his peers in the therapy groups in the prison.

William's early life was clearly difficult and damaging in terms of his development: his father walked out of the family home when William was aged 6, apparently because he had met another woman; William was always aware that there was a *'parallel family'* where he had half siblings, but his father made it clear that he was not interested in maintaining contact with William and his two younger siblings, or allowing him access to his new family. His mother struggled to manage financially, and emotionally was rather reliant on William for the first few years, confiding in him; he later described this as *'the happiest time of my life'*, even though at the time he often had to resort to stealing from shops in order for the family to eat. However, in order to make ends meet, his mother eventually took in a lodger, and quite quickly she commenced an affair with this *'handsome Yorkshire drunk'*. William's stepfather used violence to control others, and targeted all members of the family, particularly when drunk; the beatings were fearful, and William felt that he came off worst as his stepfather intended to make them cry and he refused to do so, thereby attracting vicious beatings that left him with bruises, broken ribs, and a cracked skull on one occasion. Eventually, the bruises were noticed at school, and the ensuing enquiries led to William being put into care and sent away to boarding school when he was aged 13. William described the regime there as brutal, and he was repeatedly beaten with the cane for minor misdemeanours; nevertheless, he acknowledged that he had become defiant and disruptive, having been brutalised by his experiences with his stepfather, and having learnt to adopt a provocative stance of indifference whilst inwardly struggling to control his feelings of fear.

As William left the school and entered into early adulthood, he described – with the benefit of hindsight – the way in which he vowed to himself that he would never again allow himself to feel afraid, *'to be humiliated by my fear… I became hard on the outside, never letting any challenge go, always on the attack. …[I]nside I was weak, needy and I hated it'*. He embarked on a life of acquisitive crime – theft, burglaries, and robberies – interspersed with brief periods of time in prison. In terms of relationships, William said that he longed for a family that was the opposite of his own childhood experience of family, throwing himself into relationships as a result. He acknowledged that he would idealise his partner in entirely unrealistic ways, whilst simultaneously being utterly ill-equipped for emotional commitment and steady intimacy. Each partner fell pregnant very quickly, and each baby provoked in him a feeling of terrible insecurity and jealousy as he feared the loss of his partner's love with the arrival of the child; inevitably arguments and accusations ensued, and he became disillusioned with the relationship yet tormented by fears of abandonment.

The offences of rape commenced almost by coincidence. William was in the midst of one of his burglaries and, unusually, found that he had been careless and the dwelling was occupied; when he went into the master bedroom, he found a woman asleep in the bed. He was startled and stopped, but then found himself becoming sexually aroused as he watched her and thought about her complete lack of awareness as to what was happening; he slipped his hand under the bedclothes to touch her, and in doing so, woke her up. At that point he fled the house, but he later acknowledged that at the time he ruminated on this scenario for many months, and sometimes masturbated to thoughts of the woman, although he felt *'dirty and ashamed afterwards'*. His ruminations in relation to the first incident escalated at the point his then partner left him; William described himself as *'angry ... I felt betrayed by everyone, women in particular as they were not to be trusted'*. He began to brood on the theme of revenge and to fantasise thoughts of rape during a burglary, the most exciting element of the fantasy being the feeling of total control as he noted the victim's fear and acquiescence to his demands. He prepared for rape, with a rather ritualistic approach, sourcing a knife and a balaclava mask, anticipating the scenario in his mind, and then seeking out a suitably residential neighbourhood in which to find a house to burgle. The first rape offence took place exactly as he had imagined it: his emotional state was *'stone cold, calm, focused'*; as expected, there had been no need to use the knife, and the victim had acquiesced in terror, he raped her and left the household.

William was adamant that no further rape offence took place for another year, during which time he entered a new relationship, and his partner became pregnant. However, yet again with the birth of the baby, the situation deteriorated, and following one particularly virulent argument with his partner, William started to think again about rape and planning a further assault. On this occasion, he said that he was *'more daring'* and forced the victim to perform oral sex on him, something that he felt was the ultimate expression of power; he repressed the feelings of shame that came over him afterwards, focusing instead on holding on to the intensely gratifying feelings of control that he associated with the attack, and repeatedly ruminating on the duplicity of women. The third rape took place only a few months later – again following a row during which his partner threw him out of the house. After this occasion, William began to feel afraid about his capacity to hurt a woman; he had threatened to cut the victim during the last assault and although he felt it was an empty threat at the time, the surge of rage and sexual excitement that came over him as he said it made him wonder if he had as much control over his actions as he liked to think. By this stage, the police were catching up with him, and it was with a feeling of relief that he was eventually arrested and convicted.

It took time for William to be able to face his offending, and to address his difficulties. Unlike Vic, he was confident – overly so – in a group therapy situation with other men, and he tended to dominate situations as a way of deflecting unsettling attention from himself. There were times that he was almost expelled from the therapeutic prison on account of his aggressively threatening demeanour, and it took two years before he was able to control his temper. The risk management plan had predominantly two areas of focus: learning to manage negative emotional states, particularly anger and feelings of vulnerability, and relinquishing an antisocial lifestyle. As with other men in this book with a history of institutional care and violence, William's progress was characterised by setbacks – a lapse into substance misuse, verbally threatening an offender manager, failing to declare a new intimate relationship – but there were no signs of a return to sexually aggressive fantasies or behaviour. Eventually, he made it into the community and remained there; work played a part in helping him resettle, as did a new and constructive relationship with a partner and her young daughter. Clearly, there were concerns about this at the time, and social services were closely involved in monitoring the safety of the child; but William had engaged well with his offender manager in the community, and he was able to talk through issues as they arose. The ability to offer parental care to a child who was clearly affectionate towards him was hugely rewarding for him.

Summary

I am struck, when writing about these rape narratives, of the terrible gulf between the devastating experiences of the victims and the internal world of the perpetrator. This is particularly striking with Tom and Vic, but less so for William for whom fantasy and reality were beginning to merge in a worrying escalation of behaviour. This chapter is about understanding the function of that internal world, and its relevance to any subsequent understanding of risk and treatment needs. For none of these men did pornography play a significant role, although Vic's encounter with pornography and the sexualised atmosphere of his childhood had most definitely fuelled the vibrancy of his internal world. For each of them, a common sense approach – making assumptions about sexual interests, fantasy, planning, and the offences themselves – simply did not suffice. Some of their offences were planned, others not, acts of aggression were sometimes sexually exciting but for others, something of an anticlimax or a turn off. What their differences show is that by allowing oneself to suspend judgement, and to be curious and open to new ways of thinking about violence and its precursors, it is possible to find nuance and meaning that helps us to be more effective at intervening.

Notes

1. This relates to the number of men with a sexual conviction who, after being released into the community (or on a community sentence), go on to commit a further sexual offence that comes to the attention of the authorities (that is, results in an arrest, if not a conviction).
2. This debate could equally be applied to the role of violent media in raising the risk of violent enactment, and indeed, the research findings are rather similar.
3. In which couples in a committed relationship, have an open relationship, swapping partners with other couples as a form of social activity.
4. The punishment period set by the Courts that must be spent before any consideration of release can be made by the Parole Board.

Further reading

In order to find recorded crime figures, the Office of National Statistics provides national data, and I drew on the 2019 figures:

https://www.ons.gov.uk/peoplepopulationandcommunity/crimeandjustice/articles/childsexualabuseinenglandandwales/yearendingmarch2019

There are numerous publications in relation to the downloading of child sexual abuse images. A good starting point is the work of Michael Seto, and an entire volume of *Sexual Abuse: A Journal of Research and Treatment* (2011, volume 23) is devoted to the subject.

For the reader interested in problematic online sexual behaviour, whether or not it is illegal, the following systematic reviews may be helpful:

Bothe, B., Toth-Kiraly, I., Potenza, M., Orosz, G., & Demetrovics, Z. (2020). High-frequency pornography use may not always be problematic. *Journal of Sexual Medicine*, *17*(4), 793–811.

De Alarcon, R., de la Iglesia, J., Casado, N., & Montejo, A. (2019). Online porn addiction: what we know and what we don't – a systematic review. *Journal of Clinical Medicine*, *8*(1), 91.

Mellor, E., & Duff, S. (2019). The use of pornography and the relationship between pornography exposure and sexual offending in males: a systematic review. *Aggression and Violent Behavior*, *46*, 116–126.

Finally, the UK Independent Inquiry into Child Sexual Abuse (www.iicsa.org.uk) has a wealth of information on organisations and child sexual abuse, drawing on both research evidence and expert and survivor testimony. The Internet Investigation Report (2020) provides helpful information on the use of the internet for child abuse images and child grooming offences, and can be downloaded from https://www.iicsa.org.uk/publications/investigation/internet

The practitioner's story 10

Reflecting on our emotional responses to the work

I have been asked so many times – as have my colleagues in criminal justice services – 'how do you bear it. … [D]oesn't it get to you. … I couldn't do what you do'. I recognize this sentiment, as we all have a feeling of wonder and disbelief at those who have skills or jobs in areas that seem threatening or alien to us. Nevertheless, these questions raise legitimate issues about the sustainability of work with individuals who have committed crimes that are often shocking and despicable, and who bring such an array of complexity and challenge to the core task of rehabilitation. Despondency and burn out must surely be a risk? How does one survive several decades of work in this field without falling back into self-protective strategies of indifference, cynicism, or hostile rejection? What is the emotional journey of the forensic practitioner? This chapter explores these issues, from a theoretical perspective, but also drawing on some of the personal reflections of the author after years of working with a wide range of individuals.

This book commenced with an insistence that the reader – and the practitioner – requires a stance of *curiosity* if the individual is to be understood as both representative of and yet much more than the violent offence for which he was convicted. The book now approaches the final chapter with a consideration of the role of *compassion* in enabling therapeutic and restorative work to be completed with individuals. Understanding compassion – and the obstacles to compassion that emerge during the course of the work – is central to a practitioner maintaining a healthy perspective on the work.

Understanding the nature of compassion

Accusations are commonly made that when someone expresses empathy for individuals managed by the criminal justice system – particularly those with heinous offences – they are somehow excusing the behaviour, the concern is misinterpreted as condoning; adopting a caring attitude can be seen as 'fluffy' and weak. However, as the narratives in this book have shown, it is possible to develop a deep understanding of someone and yet to hold them to account. Compassion is best understood as an evolved motivational system that has its roots in evolutionary psychology[1]: that is, compassion can be understood as *a sensitivity to suffering of self and others, with a commitment to try and alleviate and prevent it*. If we focus purely on the engagement aspects of compassion – being sensitive to cues of distress in others, managing our own feelings of distress when witnessing suffering, and having some understanding (without judgment) as to why others might be distressed – then there are risks that we may eventually burnout as a result of the persistent emotional drain that such sympathy provokes. It is engagement combined with action – behaving in a helpful way or imagining how to be helpful, and reasoning about causes and solutions, problem-solving – that makes compassion such a positive force for practitioners in the field. Interestingly, it is often the individual offender himself who struggles to show compassion to himself or to others; he too may misinterpret compassion as kindness or weakness, and feels threatened by it, rather than understanding the way in which it is linked to constructive action to change oneself and the world around one.

The premise is that those who are best able to sustain a compassionate approach to their work in criminal justice and mental health over the longer term are those who are also most able to maintain positive attitudes and high morale when working with individuals who are often extremely challenging to manage or to help change. Compassion is regularly challenged: it may be the nature of a particular crime, or the behaviour of an offender that has touched a raw nerve of a particular staff member; we can also be caught out when tired or irritable. Services draw on a range of common strategies to help maintain a healthy level of compassion in the workforce, all of which may represent common sense to the reader. For example, the role of regular supervision is to help staff reflect on their emotional responses to individual offenders and to enable them to bring greater clarity to the task at times of difficulty; and team working can diffuse the intensity of the practitioner-patient dynamic and facilitate peer support.

Box 10.1 outlines the results of an interesting research project that investigated the characteristics and behaviours that were associated with nurses who managed to maintain positive and compassionate attitudes

BOX 10.1

The attributes of staff who retain positive attitudes towards individuals with serious offences associated with pervasive personality difficulties

1. Holding a psychologically meaningful understanding of the meaning or function of behaviour that can be challenging to manage.
2. Making a set of moral choices about the importance of honesty, courage, equality, non-judgementalism, universal humanity, and individual value; and applying this to the work.
3. Engaging in a set of self-talk/thinking patterns that help one manage emotional reactions to the individuals with these convictions; this includes ways of distinguishing between the person and his offence, as he was then and is now.
4. Developing interpersonal skills, particularly in managing potentially confrontational situations, that facilitate calm and emotionally neutral responses.
5. Working as part of a team that promotes cohesion and mutual support.
6. Experiencing the organisation as supportive, in its provision of appropriate visible leadership, policies, and supervision.
7. Maintaining a compassionate stance towards the patient/client.
8. The ability to set aside negative emotional responses to behaviours and acts of violence.
9. Having clarity about the function and purpose of the service that is being delivered.

towards a very high-risk group of violent individuals with personality difficulties.[2]

The reader can see that a number of the nine traits or behaviours have featured in previous chapters in the book. Many relate to the benefits of having a meaningful theoretical model with which to understand behaviours, and to enable the separation of the act from the person; others refer to organisational structures that are supportive. Some, interestingly, relate to the personal traits of the practitioner – we might think of them as resilience factors – that involve a type of moral compass or moral reasoning that makes such practitioners particularly well-suited to the work, and more able than others to set aside their own negative emotional responses to the more challenging aspects of the work.

There are, however, times when no matter how resilient and compassionate a practitioner might be, the individual with whom we are working triggers a particular response in us that demands attention. Scattered throughout the book are narratives that touch on this feature of therapeutic working, where a reaction or a behaviour in the room – between the practitioner and the individual offender – offers a glimpse into the inner world of the individual. One of my favourite quotes that describes this beautifully is written by Richard Davies, a psychoanalyst who worked with offenders; the quote is summarised below:

> *The view is taken that professionals who deal with offenders are not free agents but potential actors who have been assigned roles in the individual offender's own re-enactment of their internal world drama. The professionals have the choice not to perform but they can only make this choice when they have a good idea of what the role is they are trying to avoid. Until they can work this out, they are likely to be drawn into the play, unwittingly, and therefore not unwillingly. Because of the latter, if the pressure to play is not anticipated then the professional will believe he is in a role of his choosing. Unfortunately, initially, only a preview of the plot is available in the somewhat cryptic form of the offence.*[3]

In Chapter 2, we referred to the structure and process of a classic detective novel as a helpful analogy for the work of a forensic practitioner; here, Davies is talking about the analogy of drama from a slightly different – but related – angle: the way in which the relationship between the individual offender and the practitioner in the room can enact or mirror early relational experiences, and perhaps even some of the dynamics of the offence itself. The practitioner's task is to be mindful of such relational dynamics – to anticipate, note, and make use of them – as they emerge. These ideas have been discussed by clinicians and therapists for decades, although probably Sigmund Freud and Anna Freud are the people most widely known for their emphasis on the unconscious and the therapist-patient relationship.[4] Box 10.2 provides some simple definitions for the key concepts – projection, transference, countertransference, and projective identification – as well as examples to try and help the reader differentiate between what are closely related and rather complex ideas.

However, one does not need to subscribe to psychoanalytic theory to acknowledge that the importance of the therapist-patient relationship has become an important component of all clinical theories in the field of mental health. Furthermore, it is absolutely central to work with those who struggle with pervasive psychological difficulties associated with their offending; see Chapter 7 for more discussion of personality disorder, and Chapter 2 for an overview of attachment theory and its importance in

BOX 10.2

Some definitions to assist with the chapter

COMPASSION

A sensitivity to suffering of self and others, with a commitment to try to alleviate and prevent it.

'I felt for him in terms of his predicament and tried to talk with him to relieve the distress he was experiencing'.

PROJECTION

A psychological defence mechanism in which a person attributes unwanted (and anxiety-provoking) thoughts, feelings, and motives onto another person rather than admitting to or dealing with the unwanted attributes.

'He insisted that his father had been good to him as a child, but I noticed that he was most prone to being violent when he perceived another man to be sneering at him, just as I felt his father had done'.

TRANSFERENCE

The unconscious process by which a person redirects feelings that s/he held in relation to key figures in childhood (often primary carers) onto an individual in adulthood, often a therapist.

'He was immediately suspicious of me as a probation officer; he seemed to think I would be just like all the other staff he had encountered as a child in care'.

COUNTERTRANSFERENCE

The unconscious or semiconscious process by which a professional or therapist redirects feelings that are held in relation to key personal figures onto the patient/client.

'I couldn't help laughing sometimes at his jokes and antics, even though I knew he was trying to distract me from the real issues in his life; I think it's because he reminded me so much of my youngest brother and the fun we had as kids together'.

PROJECTIVE IDENTIFICATION

A psychological defence mechanism in which a person attributes unwanted feelings onto another person (see Projection above) and in doing so, induces in that person the feelings that they deny within themselves.

'I found myself giving him longer sessions, running over into other people's time, because he seemed so needy, so vulnerable. I began to realise that this was a pattern in his relationships – he provoked strong maternal responses in women, and this seemed to be linked to the terrible neglect he suffered as a child. It was almost as if he could only feel cared for if others broke the rules for him, or gave him more than others received'.

understanding the layers of meaning to an offence and an individual's relational behaviour.

Of course, in reality, we are often taken unawares – Davies might say we have not read the script in advance – and find ourselves bewildered by our responses when working with complex individuals; it is by making mistakes and extricating ourselves from muddles that we learn. This is not to say that there are not occasions when the situation is simply overwhelming; no theories about unconscious processes are necessary to explain that sometimes our humanity takes over, and the nature of a particular offence is too awful to process. There are also times when despondency sets in, the task is too much, the individuals are too damaged, there is too little gratitude for the effort, the system is too intransigent; speaking personally, these are transient moments that have to be acknowledged, shared, and allowed to pass by.

The second half of this chapter is devoted to some personal reflections about moments over the past three decades that have remained with me as key learning experiences. These practitioner narratives contain elements of the unconscious processes that are outlined in Box 10.2, but also moments that have been key points on my emotional journey in the role of practitioner.

Coming down to earth with a bump

The early days of working in forensic services are characterised by a steep learning curve for many practitioners – and I include myself in this – followed by a period of what could be described as complacency: enjoying the stimulation and novelty of the work, and responding enthusiastically to friends who show an interest and want to hear about the 'stories'. Then an experience brings one up short, and makes one reflect on values and assumptions; it can be a seminal moment, a turning point.

One such seminal moment came just a few years into the work, when I became sought after as an independent expert for the first time, and asked to work on a case of sexual homicide. I was flattered and excited, keen to learn about individuals who had committed offences of the most extreme magnitude. I can still recall the moment as I sat on the train travelling to see the prisoner and reading the case file in preparation. All parole dossiers (the name given to the case file) commence with a summary account of the perpetrator, the victim, the build-up to the crime, and the details of the crime itself. These accounts can sometimes be very evocative, as it was in this case; I recall rather ancient yellowed paper – a false memory, as it was a photocopy like the rest of the dossier! – written in old-fashioned typescript from a manual typewriter (an accurate memory). The perpetrator was a man who had previous sexual convictions against children, a learning disability, and a drinking problem, and had been dreadfully abused as a child and subsequently led an itinerant and feckless life until the murder. Then I came to the short statement about the victim, which I attempt to reproduce here as an approximate version:

> *The victim, Maddy ***** was an 8-year-old girl who had been playing in the park that afternoon. She came in for her tea which was being prepared by her grandfather, who was looking after her. Tea was not yet quite ready, and so her grandfather said she could go out and play a little longer, and that she was to return in 20 minutes. She never returned, and an hour later her worried grandfather went out to look for her, and encountered the police at the crime scene.*

The perpetrator was in the park, drunk and angry about life that day; he had decided to sexually abuse a girl, and spotted Maddy returning to look for her friends. We later found out that he started to talk to her, and then touched her on the breast; she immediately responded saying *'I'm going to tell my granddaddy about you'*, looking him in the eye with a fiercely confident glare. Completely on impulse and with a burst of anger, the perpetrator picked up an old plank that was nearby and smashed it across her head.

Reading this brief outline, I was suddenly overwhelmed by the enormity of the tragedy and found myself becoming tearful on the train; my thoughts lingered on the incredible series of chance events that took place over a period of about ten minutes, that meant Maddy was in the wrong place at the wrong time, that she should have been having her tea with her grandfather, that her grandfather would live the rest of his life with the horror and regret of his decision in that moment, and that Maddy was so admirably assertive and confident in her rebuttal of the attempted abuse. There is, unfortunately, no redemptive aspect to this story: the perpetrator turned out to be utterly bewildered by his situation and seemingly unable to shift from his position as a victim of circumstances and of the system; he had had an appalling life and was both unloved and unlovable, forever alone in life and unable to move on. Two years later, I asked his solicitor how he was doing, and she said that he had had a stroke a few months earlier and then died in prison. It was the most unremittingly depressing story I had yet encountered in the work and a salutary experience for me. From that point on, although I was in no way deterred, the experience shaped my values and attitude: not only did I appreciate that glamour and excitement were a dangerous illusion, but it brought home to me how a few moments in time – with a good dose of chance and impulsive decision-making thrown in – can irrevocably transform anyone's life. Far from being thrilling, forensic work is characterised by misery and shades of grey uncertainty, rather than the black and white 'goodies' and 'baddies' of our many of our media depictions: it is really difficult to believe in pure wickedness with even the most unlikeable of perpetrators.

Being in a terrible rage

All of us in this field of work have had our moments – grinding our teeth and gripping the arms of a chair in the interview room as if our life depended on it – as we fail to deploy the best of our motivational interviewing skills, and fall back into a silent fuming anger in response to something relentlessly inappropriate that our interviewee has said. For the most part, one can wait until after the session before sharing the sense of outrage with a colleague. More often, staying alert to our emerging negative feelings provides helpful material to share with the offender in the room, when rapport has been well established: for example, raising with a man who killed his wife and who I knew quite well, '*I wonder if you notice how others respond when you talk about your wife in that sexually derogatory way? ... I find myself feeling angry on her behalf and have the impulse to defend her as she can't be here to defend herself*'. However, very occasionally, something almost visceral develops in the room so that one's negativity threatens to spill out into the session itself.

I recall one such situation, which I can only describe in terms of some sort of horror movie in which I was completely taken over by what felt like an alien – and utterly destructive – being. Clearly, the image is an extreme one, and now – even though I can recall the sensation of rage as though it were yesterday – I am struggling to think what exactly the patient had said or done to provoke such ire! The patient was an individual with very marked narcissistic traits and a history of repeated sexual offences against small children that he used to befriend in the park. I recall feeling rather smug that I had thus far resisted his provocative attempts to engage me in competitive taunts, and I had determinedly ignored his dismissal of the enormity of his actions against children. I vaguely recall that he was – at my request – attempting to put forward his account of his most recent offence; he described the 3-year-old girl victim that he had hoisted onto his shoulders in the utmost contemptuous and derogatory terms as *'sexually arousing herself'* – and thereby 'inciting' him to sexual acts that he was otherwise trying to avoid. I felt a wave of rage pass through me, and could not refrain from shouting something at him along the lines of *'but she was a 3-year-old girl having a fun ride …'* in the strident tone of someone saying 'you f***ing pervert'; although I'm almost certain I did not say this, I felt it so loudly I was sure that he must have heard.

After the session – which had ended with some mild acrimony – I lay on the clinic room floor, physically drained, and all week I brooded on my loss of control and my inappropriate response to the client. I expected a complaint, and anticipated our next session with concern: however, he appeared as normal, and made no mention of the previous week, until I felt compelled to raise, in some trepidation, *'our heated argument last week'*. He looked blank, and asked *'what argument?'* I laughed. Such a lesson for me: what to me had felt like one of the most seriously inappropriate responses I had ever made to an offender was nothing to him, he was impervious. I realised then that something in the therapist-patient relationship (see Box 10.2) did not exactly come from me or belong to me. Although I do not recall his entire history, I do remember that the individual was an unloved and isolated only child who had found solace in experiences of sexual play with other young children as he was growing up, and had coped with life by developing an impenetrable narcissistic shield around himself. All those aspects of himself that he hated – and believed that others hated about him – were projected into other people by him, and then despised. Something about my failure to respond as he expected others to respond – with immediate antagonism – may have provoked a degree of anxiety in him – unrecognised by either of us – that ultimately resulted in him needling me in order to provoke the necessary reaction. Having achieved his unconscious aim with such resounding success, all his anxiety dissipated, as I was left to deal with the corrosive remains.

Finding the most inappropriate things funny

We often think of dark humour as providing a cathartic means of coping; this is undoubtedly true but it carries with it risks: as an analogy, think of an itch and the pleasure and relief that are associated with a quick scratch;

however, if one continues scratching, the sensation becomes painful and persistent, and the habit viewed with distaste by others. Being fleetingly inappropriate in the kitchen with trusted colleagues after a difficult session is a restorative moment, but it must be shut down before slipping into the murky arena of disrespectful and contemptuous attitudes.

I have to acknowledge that over the past 30 years I have accumulated quite a list of things that have induced outbursts of hilarity, weeping with laughter with colleagues, as we indulge in inappropriate humour from time to time....

- *'Drinking too much milk'* put forward as an insightless explanation for a further offence of indecent exposure, after two painful years of unproductive therapy
- Games with colleagues in which we choose our preferred expert for when defending ourselves in court after killing an unwanted family member
- Endless discussions about how on earth one gets rid of a dead body
- Sniggering over weird sexual practices

... and so the long and rather shameful list goes on. ... I imagine the reader is puzzling over this, not least in terms of why anyone might find these examples particularly funny. They are not funny of course, and without knowing and experiencing the intensity and complexity of the situations which provoked these outbursts, it is difficult to comprehend how mildly hysterical laughter can ease the burden of compassion. There is also no doubt that such dark humour is likely to be experienced by victims of serious crimes as offensively dismissive of their intense pain, and for these reasons, I say no more about it.

Being frightened

The reality is that forensic psychologists rarely get hurt at work; prison officers, nurses, and doctors all experience their share of assaults perpetrated by frightened and angry individuals who have had to be restrained, locked up, sectioned under the Mental Health Act, or medicated against their will. However, for those of us who rely on a verbal toolkit of skills alone, the client votes with his feet whenever he can – he simply does not turn up or refuses to talk. There is another salient truth about the work, and that is – like shutting the stable door after the horse has bolted – we turn up after the violence has already taken place, and very often, the moment has passed;

few people are indiscriminately violent, and even fewer are moved to attack those who try to help them.

Interestingly, when I think back to the rare times when I have felt frightened, two individuals come to mind, both of whom ended up with a diagnosis of autistic spectrum disorder. This is not to cast individuals with autistic traits in the violent or frightening role, but there may be something about the internal workings of these particular two autistic individuals' mind that evoked fear in others. For one of these individuals, I will say little other than I was asked to contribute to an assessment of his mental state; grabbing his file just a few minutes before I met with him, I chanced upon the police case summary of his alleged offence – a detailed forensic description of the eviscerated body of his victim – and therefore went into the interview room, ill-prepared and with the horrific image of his victim imprinted on my mind. As an aside, this is an example of why – in our role as practitioners with the task of curious engagement with the perpetrator – it is a delicate balance to hold in mind sufficient information regarding the offence to achieve objectivity, but not so much as to overwhelm. Suffice to say, this severely disturbed individual presented as what I would describe as an empty vessel, utterly blank and bereft of all signs of individuality or sense of self. Immediately I was overwhelmed with a degree of terror that was utterly out of proportion to any objective risk – we were in a highly visible space in a busy healthcare department in a secure prison – and I was only able to recover myself when I ushered him out of the room. I reflected on this experience later with colleagues, and wondered whether it was this vacant quality in the perpetrator that facilitated my fear: that is, my mind – filled with the horror of the victim's injuries – fleetingly identified with her experience in a way that incapacitated me in the room.

The second individual that comes to mind was a man who presented with fairly minor but persistent offending behaviour which comprised him intermittently grabbing the breasts or buttocks of female strangers or making extremely sexually aggressive comments to them. He was an isolated individual in his mid-30s who continued to live with a mother that he experienced as cold and unemotional; he led a bleak life with little structure or purpose, and presented to forensic services with a request for help after he had received a community sentence for one of the above incidents. I was enrolled on a forensic psychotherapy course at the time that necessitated the ongoing discussion of longer term therapy clients in the small group learning set. This man seemed an ideal candidate, and I enthusiastically embarked on some therapeutic work that encouraged him to open up in the sessions and share his internal world. Within about three sessions, I had become so fearful of him that a burly male nurse from the team had to sit outside my clinic door whilst the patient was there, and I was taking taxis to the train station home, rather than walking. How could this have come about? With the benefit of experience, I now know that my stance of unfettered curiosity and exploration of his internal state of mind unleashed a bizarre assortment of sordid and violent sexual fantasies that I sought to understand and make sense of with him; this approach had the unwanted effect of producing an ever-increasing torrent of escalating sado-masochistic fantasies and dreams that began to incorporate me as a participant (as he perceived it) or victim (as I experienced it). Subjectively, I felt a terrible fear that I would be attacked by him, again, quite out of proportion to the actual behavioural risk that he posed to women; it was as if by incorporating me into his internal fantasy world, he was infiltrating my mind so that I could not think clearly or objectively, but only experience his 'dangerousness' at an emotional level. Too inexperienced to handle the situation maturely and firmly, I discharged him from my outpatient clinic rather precipitously and with a rather lame excuse, that I suspect only enflamed the situation. Gathering my wits after his final departure, I requested assistance from a forensic psychiatrist; it was perhaps two years later – following a diagnosis of high functioning autism (sometimes referred to as Asperger's) and stabilisation on medication – that this individual settled down. During this time, although he never made any move to hurt me, the individual sent the occasional letter to the Chief Executive of the NHS trust where I worked stating that I was '*a witch and a whore*' and that he wanted to '*cut off her breasts*'.

I put this experience in the 'seminal experience' category because I have no doubt that I triggered the deterioration in the man's ability to function. This alerted me to the established but rarely acknowledged finding that individuals can get worse with psychological therapy – around 10% of clients deteriorate after such interventions – and it raised the possibility in my mind that the greater the level of psychological disturbance, the less intense the intervention should probably be; one should *do no harm*. Enthusiastically tinkering with his disordered internal world was like opening a can of worms; this is another of our counter-intuitive findings in the forensic world: in the face of complexity, less is probably more.

Being sexually aroused

This topic is one that sometimes crops up between close colleagues, and I recall such conversations taking place with a sense of disbelief and dismay as we heard about incidents or colleagues who were suspended or dismissed in response to inappropriate sexual contact taking place between practitioners and patients or prisoners. For myself, I believe that strong working relationships with trusted colleagues and a settled private life enabled me to escape the undoubted risks of overstepping the accepted boundaries of work with men who have committed seriously violent offences. What might it be that drives practitioners – who otherwise are sound professionals with good intentions – to such extremes of behaviour that they know are forbidden and which will end in their self-destruction?

The *situational context* for such sexually boundaryless behaviour tends to be intimacy – whether this is the intense intimacy of the therapy couch, or the confusing intimacy of the nurse or prison officer playing pool, or walking around the courtyard chatting with an offender who otherwise is subject to their strict controls. The *organisational context* tends to be one of problematic culture, in which staff are not encouraged to explore and reflect on the complexity of their relationships with offenders; the absence of supervision and support means that minor boundary transgressions – the amount of time spent with an individual, the way in which the practitioner dresses, the slip-ups of self-disclosure to an offender – are not picked up in time. Those *staff* who fall into catastrophic boundary transgressions are not necessarily the most naïve or inexperienced, but those who are struggling with a personal situation that renders them vulnerable to the attentions of others – loneliness, marital breakdown, geographical separation from family, financial stress. Finally, what ingredient does the *individual offender* brings to the toxic recipe? We heard from Owen in Chapter 7 that his seduction of the prison visitor was probably driven by psychopathic traits such as a rapid propensity for boredom, and a rather callous focus on the material benefits that such a relationship might offer him. However, for many men damaged by developmental experiences that provided inconsistent or anxiety-provoking weak attachments to problematic carers, drawing a practitioner into a relationship that oversteps their professional boundaries provides the ultimate indication that they are truly special, truly cared for. For some men with highly sexualised childhoods, it is the sex that provides a level of reassurance that caring or kindness could never do; for other men, it is the fact that s/he *'broke the rules for me'* that is the ultimate test of caring.

I would suggest that within the forensic context, it is more likely that a sexual breach of boundaries will take place when these four factors are present; and that it is the responsibility of the system – the organisations and professional bodies – to ensure that their duty of care to staff includes providing the supervision and training to minimise the risks of such catastrophic boundary violations.

Giving up… or on heroic attempts to repair the irreparable

We have already discussed the practitioner's need for resilience in the work, balancing an objective and cool-headed appraisal of the individual offender's risk with a compassionate and hopeful engagement in the work of rehabilitation with the same individual. Occasionally this delicate balance is challenged; most commonly, this occurs early in one's career at a time when our enthusiastic confidence in the power of kindness and therapy to reform characters who have previously been misunderstood and neglected is at its height! Having been there myself, I recognise this state of mind in my more junior colleagues and watch with dismay as their rather idealistic hopes buckle in the face of disappointment and failure. The key task – if one wants to persist with the work –for a practitioner is to learn to accept the bumpy nature of the redemptive path, and that therapeutic relationships are something of a long haul, with ups and downs (the latter often involving a return to prison). Adapting to this new and more modest aspiration for the work facilitates a longer term resilience. Having successfully navigated this stage in my career, I was a seasoned practitioner, with what I would consider to be a clear-eyed vision of my work with challenging clients, when I first found myself absolutely and utterly 'giving up' with a man under my care. This state of giving up was an emotional one – no one would necessarily have noticed it in me – but I knew at that moment of despair that I had lost any capacity for useful engagement with him.

I recall the final straw with great clarity. This man had been most horribly abused, neglected, and misunderstood as a child, and his subsequent behaviour had alienated his hostile family environment still further. On four separate occasions he had been sentenced for the sexual abuse of pubescent boys: probation officers had stopped putting him on sex offender treatment programmes, the police wanted him back inside prison, housing refused to offer him a permanent flat, and he was turned down for disability benefit despite very obvious physical health problems. Now aged 59 – but looking as though he was 70 or more – he was referred to me for the third time, as he vacillated to and fro from prison to a bedsit in the community. Although he had not committed a sexual offence for 15 years, he latched on to neighbours and local church goers in his loneliness and in doing so, regularly ignored the strict rules that forbade him from speaking to anyone under the age of 18. I had tried everything from therapy to medication, to obtaining him a better flat, and volunteer support. He was dependent and needy, engaged in problematic behaviours that spoke more of habit and isolation rather than a strong drive to sexually offend. It was within this context that we found ourselves talking about the seaside one day – triggered by some item in the news – and he spoke longingly of how he had never seen the sea or felt the sand between his toes (although his siblings had been to the coast) because he had never lived in a family environment where anyone felt he deserved a treat. Somehow the idea of a visit to the seaside became a focus of all that was wrong in his life, a symbol of his deprivation; over time, his volunteer support worker proposed taking him on a trip for a 'treat', but key agencies were opposed to the idea because of his offending history. I found myself latching on to his sense of longing, fighting his corner with a slightly surprising degree of conviction and zeal, first with probation and then with police, organising travel funds and so on.

Despite my exhaustion at all this effort, it was with great anticipation that I awaited the man's feedback after the trip; I think I hoped that he would have experienced some wistful pleasure tinged with sadness, bringing some emotional material that we might be able to think about together. He arrived at our session and reported in a rather flat tone of voice that the seaside *'was alright but it rained a bit and I never got to buy a stick of rock'*, then moving on to complain about several other matters relating to his benefits and his broken fridge, that indicated how he was continuously being let down by others. And that was that! As though a light had been switched off, I gave up completely and disengaged emotionally from him. I realised that his level of psychological damage was such that he had defeated me, and nothing that I did could in any way repair the ways in which he was broken; it was like pouring water endlessly into a colander and watching it constantly leaking all the water out through the holes. Now I can look back and reflect more calmly on the ways in which I was forced to experience his unbearable inner state of being at an emotional, rather than purely cerebral, level; but this insight does not change the fact that every practitioner has their compassion limits, and I had met mine on that day.

Getting it wrong

What does it feel like to use all one's skills as a practitioner to assess the risk that a man poses to others and to believe that risk to be low; to engage him in meaningful therapeutic work to keep that risk to a minimum; to believe that all the evidence suggests he is making positive progress; and yet, to find that has lied during sessions and has committed a catastrophically violent offence in-between two of those sessions?

In some ways, this book has been about deception as well as hope: personal narratives of men who have been let down, and who learn to turn the tables in order to ensure that they are never again duped about matters that make them feel vulnerable. This includes perceptions of deception in relation to things not being what they seem, parents faking love, professionals mimicking concern, prisoners lying about their offending behaviour, adults pretending to love when actually they abuse to meet their own needs, offenders asking for help but have no intention of actually making use of that help when offered, society pretending to hold values of social inclusion but pursuing a line of 'not in my backyard'. It is perhaps inevitable that the practitioner has to experience something of the deception that the individual offender has experienced, and in doing so come to know what it feels like to be duped. Lesser forms of deception can be tolerated and thought about – 'small' lies and acts of omission – but the great fear of any forensic practitioner is to be deceived in relation to risk and reoffending. Believing someone to be high risk who subsequently reoffends simply confirms the accuracy of one's risk assessment; in such circumstances, the practitioner hopes to feel that at least they did everything they could to reduce the risk by the means available to them. Believing someone to be high risk and they turn out not to reoffend is a pleasant surprise, and one that builds learning and confidence. However, the great fear is that one believes someone to be low risk, and they commit a grave offence that causes devastation to the victims whilst under our care or supervision.

The story of professional failure that I have chosen to share – albeit in sketchy outline – is the case of a man who was convicted of Wounding with intent to cause Grievous Bodily Harm some 30 years before I knew him, and who served an indeterminate sentence before eventually being released by the Parole Board. He had very seriously assaulted a man during the course of a casual sexual encounter in which bondage and other sado-masochistic activities had taken place. Every care had been taken to ensure that his risk had been addressed during the sentence, and progression to the community was very cautiously undertaken with a good deal of testing at each stage. He was, at the time, my most motivated and reflective outpatient in the community, with considerable insight into his previous offence and the contributory factors; he had a superb probation officer managing his supervision, with whom he had a strong working relationship. We had been concerned a few weeks prior to the incident, when his mood appeared to dip in response to a very humiliating rejection by a charity for whom he had expected to be able to volunteer – he spoke vividly at the time of the manager's appalled response when reading the man's disclosure letter[5] – but with our support and encouragement, he seemed to rally and recoup his former hopefulness regarding reintegration into the community. I was due to meet with him the next day for a routine appointment, and it was therefore a devastating shock to me when I received a call from the police to say that he was at the station, having made an attempt to hang himself prior to being charged with attempted murder. It emerged that he had bought a knife and rope and had gone out into the street and attacked a female stranger; if it had not been for the intervention of her friend who was nearby, she may well have died from her injuries.

This story, selfishly, is not about the terrible impact of the attack on the victim herself, or on her friend, both of whom in their different ways were likely to have been absolutely traumatised by the experience. The focus of the narrative is on the impact on the practitioner when such events occur, no matter how rare the event. Although I can confidently state that such an experience has almost never occurred on my watch – that I, as with most forensic practitioners, have striven to ensure that my work keeps the public safe – this makes no difference to how personally one interprets the failure. In this case, the subsequent impersonal machinery of reviews and investigations found that both I and the probation officer had provided very good care and supervision, but this too made little difference. For a conscientious practitioner, the aftermath of a serious incident feels persecutory no matter with what care and kindness the investigation is conducted. We each responded in different ways: for the probation officer, when I spoke to him later, the impact was to shatter his belief in his judgement and his professionalism, the key fact being that he had never seen this coming, and he resigned from the service three months later. My own reaction was to be equally shocked, but my response was to become utterly preoccupied with trying to understand what had happened and why; it felt as though I did not sleep for a month, although this is an exaggeration, and every night I would feel compelled to go through the build-up to the new offence – or what I knew of it – in pedantic and repetitive detail in my mind. This may feel familiar to those who have suffered an unexpected traumatic event and find themselves repeatedly seeking information and answers in order to process the experience and – ultimately – to put it to rest in some way. For me, I was only able to move on after I went to visit the man in prison and talk to him about what had happened. His account was that the trigger for this attack was that his probation session the day before had enraged him, because his probation officer had had to convey the news that his manager had refused to reduce his risk level from high to medium just yet, stating that it was too soon. Objectively, this was not necessarily an unreasonable position for the manager to hold, nor did it have any observably negative consequences for the man's progress in the community; however, he experienced it as somehow negating his humanity, his efforts to progress, and as persecutory and authoritarian. With hindsight, it is possible to see how this session may have reignited his feelings of humiliation and rejection at the hands of the potential employer a few weeks earlier. His response was to think *'if they think I'm high risk, I'll show them what high risk is'*; he said that he brooded all night, and then determined to commit another offence. The next day, he left the flat, and noted his relapse prevention plan – pinned to the inside of his front door – stated 'in a crisis ring Jackie' but he ignored it and left to commit the offence.

It would not be true to say that his narrative made total sense to me, although I recognised the sentiment that other offenders or ex-offenders have expressed: 'no matter how many programmes or how many rules you make me comply with, whether or not I reoffend is entirely a matter of my choice'. However, the act of enquiry and the development of his story enabled me to process the experience, and take what learning I could from it.

Concluding remarks

This experience of professional failure, with its devastating consequences, is perhaps a dismal note on which to conclude this chapter on the practitioner's narrative. However, I would prefer to suggest that it provides a note of caution and realism, rather than despair. The practitioner's task is always to seek to adopt a compassionate approach to working with men whose seriously violent offending behaviour is driven by motives that are sometimes explicit but more often obscured from view and overlaid with complexity. In order to be able to sustain the work – and as importantly remain motivated and enthused by the work – it is important to bring some realism and humility to the task. The vignettes in this chapter are personal reminiscences of some of the learning points in my forensic career; other practitioners may recognise aspects of my shared experiences but will also have a myriad of stories that reflect their own pathway to learning and building resilience.

This book was initially conceived as a means of responding to the many questions that curious colleagues and friends posed when seriously violent offences were the topic of conversation, the themes being repeated again and again. 'Surely some crimes are motiveless, does evil exist, how does an experience of sexual abuse as a child translate into becoming a perpetrator in adulthood, what is personality disorder, is he a psychopath, I was in care and I haven't gone on to hurt other people, if you look at indecent images of children you must be a paedophile, how do you know he's low risk now when he was capable of such violence? ...' and so on. Good questions, and a necessary first step to developing an understanding. Formulating an answer has always been an interesting challenge, and I have chosen here to explain by means of the individuals' narratives, as facts and figures – as I have learned – make little impression as compared to the humanity of a person's story. Hearing these stories – really listening with an open mind to what is being conveyed – is the responsibility of the reader. My hope is that these stories have helped the interested reader to move from a position of comfortable moral certainty to a slightly less comfortable position of moral complexity or ambiguity. Right and wrong has not changed because behaviour that harms others is personally and socially unacceptable and we endorse the role of punishment as an expression of this condemnation for wrongdoing. However, perhaps good and bad is not so black and white: for example, some of these men's narratives seem to suggest it is possible to commit a horrendous offence and yet demonstrate courage in exposing one's most personal vulnerabilities and turning one's life around; others raise questions of shared culpability when perpetrators have faced such unacknowledged adversity and abuse as children that their pathways into adulthood have, at the very least, been contaminated.

In bringing this narrative to a close, I want to restate the task of the forensic practitioner as one that needs to be shared with the society in which we work: it is a precarious balance to maintain curiosity and compassion for the offender side with the rightful expectations of society that it be kept safe from harm.

Notes

1. Evolutionary psychology is a theoretical approach that considers key psychological traits or concepts as having a meaningful function in relation to natural selection.
2. Bowers, L. (2002). *Dangerous and Severe Personality Disorder: Response and Role of the Psychiatric Team*. New York: Routledge.
3. Davies, R. (1996). The inter-disciplinary network and the internal world of the offender. In (eds.) C. Cordess & M. Cox, *Forensic Psychotherapy: Crime, Psychodynamics and the Offender Patient* (pp. 133–144). London: Jessica Kingsley. Extract from page 133.
4. For an accessible book on psychodynamic ideas in this area, Malan, D. (2007) *Individual Psychotherapy and the Science of Psychodynamics*, 2nd edition. London: Hodder Arnold.
5. An important but difficult component of rigorous risk management in the community is the expectation that offenders on probation supervision – in this case, life licence – disclose sufficient detail of their offending history for a potential employer to make an informed decision about risk.

Index